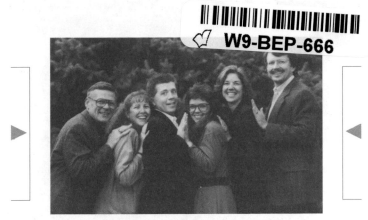

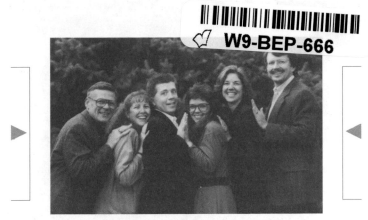

Our "Compacted" Compact Clinicals Team

Dear Valued Customer,

WELCOME to Compact Clinicals. We are committed to bringing mental health professionals up-to-date diagnostic and treatment information in a compact, timesaving, and easy-to-read format. Our line of books provides current, thorough reviews of assessment and treatment strategies for mental disorders.

We've "compacted" complete information for diagnosing each disorder and comparing how different theoretical orientations approach treatment. Our books use nonacademic language, real-world examples, and well-defined terminology.

Enjoy this and other timesaving books from Compact Clinicals.

Sincerely,

Melanie Dean, Ph.D.
President

Compact Clinicals Line of Books

Compact Clinicals currently offers these condensed reviews for professionals:

For Clinicians

Attention Deficit Hyperactivity Disorder
The latest assessment and treatment strategies

C. Keith Conners, Ph.D.

Bipolar Disorder
The latest assessment and treatment strategies

Trisha Suppes M.D., Ph.D., and Ellen B. Dennehy, Ph.D.

Borderline Personality Disorder
The latest assessment and treatment strategies

Melanie Dean, Ph.D.

Conduct Disorders
The latest assessment and treatment strategies

J. Mark Eddy, Ph.D.

Depression in Adults
The latest assessment and treatment strategies

Anton Tolman, Ph.D.

Obsessive Compulsive Disorder
The latest assessment and treatment strategies

Gail Steketee, Ph.D., and Teresa Pigot, M.D.

Post-Traumatic and Acute Stress Disorders
The latest assessment and treatment strategies

Matthew Friedman, M.D., Ph.D.

For Physicians

Bipolar Disorder: Treatment and Management

Trisha Suppes, M.D., Ph.D., and Paul E. Keck, Jr., M.D.

Attention Deficit Hyperactivity Disorder

The latest assessment and treatment strategies

Third Edition

C. Keith Conners, Ph.D.

Juliet L. Jett, Ph.D., Contibuting Author

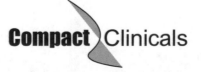

Attention Deficit Hyperactivity Disorder

The latest assessment and treatment strategies

Third Edition

by

C. Keith Conners, Ph.D.

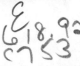

Compact Clinicals

Published by: Compact Clinicals
7205 NW Waukomis Dr., Suite A
Kansas City, MO 64151

816-587-0044

©2006 Dean Psych Press Corp. d/b/a Compact Clinicals
Prior Releases: ©1999, 2001 by C. Keith Conners, Ph.D. and Juliet L. Jett, Ph.D.

Medical Editing: Kathi L. Whitman, In Credible English, Inc.,®
Kansas City, Missouri

Book Design: Coleridge Design, Kansas City, Missouri

Library of Congress Cataloging in Publication data:

Conners, C. Keith
Attention Deficit Hyperactivity Disorder : the latest assessment and treatment strategies / by C. Keith Conners.—[3rd]
        p.   ; cm.
    Includes bibliographical references and index.
    ISBN 13: 978–1-887537-23-0
    ISBN 10: 1-887537-23-6
    1. Attention-deficit hyperactivity disorder. 2. Attention deficit-disordered children. 3. Attention-deficit disorder in adults. I. Title.
    RJ506.H9C648 2006
    618.92'8589–dc22
        2005008627

10 9 8 7 6 5 4 3 2 1

Read Me First

As a mental health professional, often the information you need can only be obtained after countless hours of reading or library research. If your schedule precludes this time commitment, Compact Clinicals is the answer.

Our books are practitioner oriented with easy-to-read treatment descriptions and examples. Compact Clinicals books are written in a nonacademic style. Our books are formatted to make the first reading, as well as ongoing reference, quick and easy. You will find:

- ► **Anecdotes** — Each chapter contains a fictionalized account that personalizes the disorder entitled, "From the Patient's Perspective."

- ► **Sidebars** — Narrow columns on the outside of each page highlight important information, preview upcoming sections or concepts, and define terms used in the text.

- ► **Definitions** — Terms are defined in the sidebars where they originally appear in the text and in an alphabetical glossary on pages 89 through 92.

- ► **References** — Numbered references appear in the text following information from that source. Full references appear on pages 93 through 106.

- ► **Case Examples** — Our examples illustrate typical client comments or conversational exchanges that help clarify different treatment approaches. Identifying information in the examples (e.g., the individual's real name, profession, age, and/or location) has been changed to protect the confidentiality of those clients discussed in case examples.

- ► **Key Concepts** — At the end of each chapter, we include a review list of key concepts from that chapter. Use these lists for ongoing quick reference as well as for reviewing what you learned from reading the chapter.

Contents

Chapter One:
Overview of ADHD

This chapter answers the following:

► **How Common is ADHD?** — This section presents prevalence rates among children and adults.

► **What are the "Knowns" and "Unknowns" of ADHD?** — This section reviews those areas that reflect consensus as well as those that reflect disagreement in our current knowledge about the disorder. This section discusses core symptoms about which researchers seem to agree.

► **Will Children with ADHD "Grow Out of It?"** — This section highlights research on whether those with ADHD will continue experiencing symptoms through adolescence and into adulthood.

ATTENTION Deficit Hyperactivity Disorder (ADHD) is one of the most commonly diagnosed mental disorders of children, accounting for 30 to 40 percent of all referrals made to child guidance clinics as well as pediatric, family, and primary care practices. In addition, this same disorder accounts for a significant percentage of recent referrals in adult treatment settings.

This chronic mental disorder begins early in life and has a characteristic symptom picture and developmental course throughout the lifespan. ADHD symptoms typically impair social, educational, or occupational functioning across multiple settings and are not caused by other mental disorders.

Many children are either over-diagnosed or under-diagnosed, often due to the disorder's developmental nature and concerns about inappropriately medicating children experiencing what may be normal behavior for their age and gender. Just as clinicians evaluate height and body weight in relation to the age and gender of normal children, so ADHD symptoms must be judged in relation to the age and sex of normal children. Thus, the hyperactivity of a normal five-year-old boy may be significantly higher than the restless, hyperactive behavior of a normal, 10-year-old boy, and a child diagnosed with ADHD must differ significantly from these norms.

The Diagnostic and Statistical Manual of Mental Disorders (DSM) has historically considered hyperactivity (or impulsivity) the key feature of an ADHD diagnosis. The latest edition, DSM-IV (TR), now lists prominent hyperactive-impulsive symptoms as a subtype of the disorder.[1]

I

How Common is ADHD?

ADHD prevalence statistics come from research studies with conflicting results, usually traced to differences in the study criteria. For example, several studies reported that two to five percent of school-aged children have well-defined and pervasive symptoms of ADHD, which translates into a prevalence rate of between 1,000,000 and 3,000,000 children suffering from the disorder at any point in time.[2-6]

However, other research indicates that many children are diagnosed and given medications who do not in fact qualify for the diagnosis, and many others are not being diagnosed by practitioners in the community and treated appropriately.[7]

Child referral sources may pay more attention to boys than girls because they appear to be more aggressive, irritable, and likely to interrupt others. On the other hand, adults seeking treatment may be more concerned with their attention, organizational skills, and memory.

There is evidence that ADHD prevalence in children also relates to gender differences and preferences of child referral sources. Although researchers estimate that boys are three to 10 times more affected with the disorder than girls, self-referred adults appear to be equally affected.[8, 9]

The amount of recent scientific and lay literature has led to a rapid increase in ADHD diagnosis among adults as well. Prevalence estimates vary widely, depending on the criteria used to define a case; however, those studies that use rigorous diagnoses, clear measures of impairment, and careful differential diagnosis indicate a prevalence rate of two to four percent.[7]

What Are the "Knowns" and "Unknowns" of ADHD?

Although ADHD is a common mental disorder and has been recognized in one form or another for over a century, researchers and clinicians still cite many unknown aspects of the disorder.

Those who suffer from ADHD typically present symptoms grouped as either related to inattentiveness, hyperactivity/impulsivity, or to a combination of both.

> ▶ **Symptoms of inattentiveness** include making careless mistakes and being disorganized as well as having trouble listening to others, following instructions, or completing tasks. Children with ADHD often avoid tasks that require prolonged attention, are forgetful, and can be easily distracted during activities.

> ▶ **Symptoms of hyperactivity and impulsiveness** include being restless and fidgety as well as intruding on others. Children with these ADHD symptoms tend to speak out of turn by butting into conversations or blurting out comments inappropriately. In addition, they have trouble being patient and/or playing quietly.

What We Know

- ▶ How to define core ADHD symptoms of hyperactivity, impulsivity, and inattentiveness
- ▶ What are commonly associated features of ADHD
- ▶ How common ADHD is among children
- ▶ That the disorder continues into adulthood

What We Don't Know

- ▶ The exact symptom criteria for defining ADHD
- ▶ How severe symptoms must be to diagnose the disorder
- ▶ What level of functional impairment by age and gender is symptomatic of ADHD
- ▶ How to resolve the conflicting evidence regarding the disorder's origin
- ▶ How the disorder changes over time and presents itself in adulthood
- ▶ What treatments and treatment combinations are most effective at various ages and for various symptoms and degrees of symptom severity, especially for the more complex cases with many comorbid symptoms
- ▶ What genetic or other kinds of subtypes exist within the broad pool of ADHD patients
- ▶ How to best define impairment criteria

ADHD's different presentations make it difficult for experts to define the disorder. In fact, continuing controversy exists as to whether ADHD is one disorder or a spectrum of different disorders. Our understanding has changed radically over time, with definitions varying between a disorder with a neurobiological basis and one caused by environment and social learning.

Much of the controversy regarding diagnosis comes from failure to adhere to recommended guidelines. However, evidence shows that the disorder can be reliably diagnosed when diagnostic criteria are carefully followed, using:[10]

- ▶ Expert guidelines [11–13]
- ▶ Practice parameters recommended by the American Academy of Child and Adolescent Psychiatry[14]
- ▶ *Normed rating scales*[15] (see chapter two)

In the past, clinicians have characterized the disorder as "organic drivenness," "minimal brain dysfunction," "hyperkinetic syndrome," "attention deficit disorder," and (most recently) "attention deficit hyperactivity disorder." Although the current description is expressed in purely behavioral terms, scientific evidence strongly suggests a biological basis for the underlying causes, but with significant environmental factors that impact the dis-

normed rating scales — assessment tools, validated against a normal population, that measure symptom severity at different developmental periods, such as childhood, adolescence, and adulthood.

genetic transmission — the transmission of chromosomal links, which influence the development of an organism from one generation to another

ease.[1, 16–18] These causes include *genetic transmission*, personality or temperament, prenatal and postnatal factors, brain structure differences, and possible brain chemical differences.[17, 19–26] Lead in the environment, second-hand cigarette smoke, alcohol use during pregnancy, and various extreme environments (such as trauma, neglect, or abuse in childhood) can produce symptoms that mimic those of ADHD. Maternal use of cigarettes during pregnancy is one of the stronger risk factors.[27]

Various biological and environmental risk factors interact to produce ADHD.[19, 28–31] For example, someone with a genetic tendency toward a high activity level might be in a high-stress family environment, which would increase the likelihood of having ADHD. Conversely, there may be a variety of protective factors in the family, which keep appearance of the disorder below the level of impairment, such as: high IQ, good economic resources, strong social skills, excellent individualized schooling, or a positive family environment.[32, 35] This *risk model* approach helps to resolve much of the conflicting evidence regarding ADHD origins, since several small risks (as well as a single, strong risk factor) can combine to produce the same outcomes.[34]

risk model — conceptualization of a disease based on an accumulation of risks that increases the likelihood of a particular disorder emerging

Will Children with ADHD "Grow Out of It"?

Good evidence exists that those with ADHD continue to have problems through adolescence and even as adults, though the exact manner in which the symptoms appear may change. Adolescents and adults tend to exhibit more symptoms related to self-esteem, competence, family functioning, managing interpersonal relationships, and anger control.[35, 36]

Chapter two reviews common difficulties experienced by those with ADHD throughout their lifespan, including those typical of adolescents and adults, as well as the latest research on diagnostic criteria differences for adults.

Recent studies of symptoms in adult and adolescent ADHD indicate a greater emphasis on cognitive symptoms and problems with self-esteem than is reported in childhood.[35]

Researchers estimate that 30 to 50 percent of adults diagnosed with ADHD during childhood will continue to have problems and will report symptoms acute enough to cause impairment in daily functioning.[37] Often, adults with ADHD make frequent job changes and demonstrate poor work performance. Additionally, they tend to feel impatient, perceive tasks as repetitive and uninteresting over time, and feel restless or bored.

According to recent, long-term studies, only about 75 percent of these adults graduate from high school, and very few complete college. Although they are as likely to be employed as those without ADHD, their work status tends to be lower, associated to some extent with their lower level of education.[38] ADHD sufferers also engage in more premarital sex, give birth to more children outside marriage, and have more sexually-transmitted diseases than their normal peers.[39]

Studies of young adults with ADHD (ages 18 to 22) indicate no overall differences in employer ratings of work performance or frequency of employment compared to others. However, those with the disorder experienced more frequent job changes, worked several part-time jobs, and became dissatisfied more easily as time went on. After several years of employment, employers rated work performance for those with ADHD as inferior in certain areas, such as completing tasks and working independently. However, employer ratings of punctuality and good working relationships remained similar to non-ADHD workers. The results from this study also indicate no significant difference in average annual income despite changes in work performance over time.[37]

Some mental disorders are more prevalent among adults with ADHD, especially antisocial personality disorder and substance abuse disorders, occurring much more frequently in those experiencing inattention, impulsivity, and hyperactivity.

Those who fail to show continued impairment as adults and function well in their daily environment may do so for a number of reasons. Symptoms may remit over time, ending the disruptive influence and impairment. Environmental changes that occur when someone transitions from student to working adult may also play a part, since home and work environments can be more varied for adults than children.

Adult choices can be timed to individual needs, rather than to the schedule of a parent or teacher.

One study found a much higher percentage of those with childhood ADHD managing their own businesses.[38] This could result from these peoples' ability to utilize unique skills and energies, or it could result from their difficulty in relating to authority and working for others.

From the Patient's Perspective

Mom is taking me to see some doctor today. I guess I'm getting on her nerves lately. It doesn't help that I broke that lamp yesterday. It sure bugs her when I don't listen and don't finish things I start. Seems like those other kids can pay attention a whole lot better than me. Sometimes I just don't get what the teacher is talking about because I can't stand having to sit still and do nothing. Maybe this doctor can help me do better at school.

Key Concepts for Chapter One:

1. ADHD is a chronic mental disorder that typically begins early and follows a developmental pattern throughout one's life.

2. Although prevalence rates for ADHD vary due to gender differences and child referral sources, recent estimates are two to five percent for children and two to four percent for adults.

3. The disorder can be reliably diagnosed using expert guidelines, practice parameters set by the American Academy of Child and Adolescent Psychiatry, and normed rating scales.

4. ADHD appears to result from the interaction of varied biological and environmental risk factors.

5. In adolescents and adults, ADHD appears to cause more problems with thinking and self-esteem than in childhood.

Chapter Two:
Diagnosing and Assessing ADHD

This chapter answers the following:

▶ **What are Typical Characteristics of Those with ADHD?** — This section discusses ADHD symptoms present at different developmental stages, from infancy to adulthood.

▶ **What are the Specific DSM-IV (TR) Criteria for Diagnosing ADHD?** — This section features a reprint of current DSM-IV (TR) criteria for diagnosing ADHD as well as important clarifying information.

▶ **What Assessment Techniques Can Be Used to Diagnose ADHD?** — This section covers interview techniques, observation techniques, and psychometric assessment tools.

▶ **What Differentiates ADHD from other Disorders?** — This section presents disorders or symptom areas that must be differentiated from ADHD for accurate diagnosis.

DIAGNOSING ADHD requires a careful assessment process that uses varying information, depending on the purpose of the diagnosis. A diagnostic purpose of developing a comprehensive treatment plan requires much more assessment data than one required for purely administrative reasons.

Factors involved in diagnosing ADHD significantly influence the thoroughness of the assessment process in the following ways:

▶ **Need to classify someone as eligible for special services** — Formal diagnosis (according to criteria set forth in the DSM-IV) is used to determine which patients qualify for special services, reimbursement by managed care, and participation in clinical research studies.

▶ **Need to determine a course of treatment** — A treatment plan goes beyond what is required for formal classification. In addition to verifying that symptoms presented meet established criteria for diagnosis, an assessor collects enough detail to determine which treatments are needed, how and when they are implemented, and what the future course of the disorder is likely to be. These cases require assessment of the family, academic, social, and physical environment. This is the only kind of meaningful assessment in a clinical context that is appropriate for treating and managing ADHD.

▶ **Need to plan for treatment monitoring** — Because treatments initiated after diagnosis require close monitoring, the information gathered during the assessment process needs to include specific types and frequency of impaired functioning at school, home, on the job, in social relationships, and in personality functioning. This

prognosis — outcome in
the future

information provides a baseline against which treatment progress and developmental change can be measured.

▶ **Need to link treatment to *prognosis*** — Because many factors may influence the course and outcome of the disorder, including family psychiatric history, exposure to certain environmental elements, and family functioning or adversity, the assessment process should gather this information to determine appropriate treatment. In turn, the treatments selected will impact the outcome.

Whatever the diagnostic purpose, assessment must focus on symptoms in light of age and developmental level. The symptoms of ADHD must occur at a level that is developmentally inappropriate, because many normal people have similar symptoms. Therefore, the symptoms must occur more often than the norm for children and adults of the same age.

DSM-IV (TR) — the leading
diagnostic guide for mental
disorders (**Diagnostic and
Statistical Manual of
Mental Disorders, Fourth
Edition, Text Revision**,
published by the American
Psychiatric Association)

DSM-IV (TR) requires symptoms causing impairment to be present by the age of seven. However, there is doubt about the validity of this age requirement, and clinicians should consider that, although the basic pattern may be evident at any age, its onset is considered to be "early," which means occurring in either the preschool or school-age child.[40]

What are Typical Characteristics of Those with ADHD?

inattention — brief attention
focus that is often frustrating
to others

distractability — stimuli
in the environment attracts
attention away from the task
at hand

impulsivity/hyperactivity
— acting without thinking,
often putting the person at risk

The key characteristics associated with ADHD are: *inattention*, *distractibility*, and *impulsivity/hyperactivity*, as well as an inability to fit in with peers. Figure 2.1, on the next page, presents illustrative behaviors in children and adults.

Symptoms appearing for the first time in adolescence or adulthood may reflect some other disorder, such as depression or anxiety. However, some children may not have exhibited ADHD symptoms in childhood because various protective factors masked the disorder. Research indicates that family and parental problems heighten the risk for disorder, whereas being a good student, getting along with others, and participating in extra-curricular activities reduce the risk.[41]

Although primary ADHD symptoms can occur at all ages, certain symptoms are more prominent during certain age spans and developmental levels .

Figure 2.1 Typical ADHD Behavior

	In Children	In Adults
Inattention	• Needing the teacher to give instructions repeatedly • Playing with five or six different games or toys within the same period other children play with a single game or toy	• Acting disinterested or avoiding activities requiring sustained attention, such as watching movies, reading, painting, or sewing
Distractibility	• Taking out the trash but getting distracted along the way by the dog, a younger brother, a toy, and something interesting in the trash, resulting in never making it to the outside trash bin	• Never finishing tasks when interrupted
Impulsivity/ Hyperactivity	• Being up, down, and all over a chair while watching television • Interrupting somebody while they are talking • Running into the street without looking • Jumping from a roof because it "looked fun" • Engaging in nonstop motor activity and being more restless than normal children while sleeping (younger children)[3]	• Buying on impulse or making "on-the-spot" decisions without thinking through the consequences
Inability to Fit in with Peers	• Not waiting for a turn • Not following rules (although they are known and understood) in social situations	• Having trouble getting along with coworkers or changing jobs frequently due to disagreements with employers

ADHD as a Developmental Disorder

ADHD has important developmental features, beginning possibly as early as infancy and continuing in various forms throughout the lifespan.

Symptoms may be expressed differently at different developmental periods. Some symptoms, such as restlessness, may be experienced by adolescents or adults as internal restlessness or discomfort rather than overt behavior when in situations requiring them to remain seated or still (e.g., in a classroom or business meeting). Research shows that the overt hyperactive-impulsive behaviors tend to wane in older children and adults, whereas inattentive symptoms tend to remain or become more obvious.

Although ADHD is not formally diagnosed in infancy, children who receive an informal diagnosis as young as age two tend to retain the same diagnosis at school age.[42] One study reported that parents of approximately one-third of the children diagnosed with ADHD remembered difficulties with excessive crying, sleep and feeding problems, and disturbed interactive behaviors. For instance, many parents described their children during infancy as:[37]

▶ Crying frequently and being difficult to soothe

▶ Having sleep disturbances such as being excessively

Figure 2.2, on the next page, summarizes this changing pattern of symptoms and impairments from one developmental stage to another. The text that follows figure 2.2 details typical symptoms related to each developmental stage with some discussion of research on infant presentation.

Figure 2.2   ADHD Symptoms and Developmental Stages

Characteristic Symptoms	
Preschool	• Destructive with toys and household items • Excitable • Hyperactive (child is always on the go or described as "driven by a motor"; climbs on and gets into things constantly) • Fidgety • Noisy • Aggressive • Stubborn (low level of compliance, especially with boys) • Temper tantrums (that far exceed those of "normal" children in frequency, severity, and duration) • Accident prone • Insatiable curiosity • Demanding of parental attention • Difficulty completing developmental tasks (such as toilet training) • Decreased and/or restless sleep • Delays in motor or language development • Family difficulties (including obtaining and keeping baby sitters, especially with children with severe problems)
Middle Childhood	• Easily distracted from tasks • Hyperactive • Poorly organized; engages in off task activities • Fails to complete homework and other projects • Disruptive in class; acts like class clown • Bored all the time • Interrupts • Can't wait turn • Impulsive • Displays aggression • Has increasing difficulty with peer relationships
Adolescence	• Daydreams • Poorly organized; poor follow-through • Restless • Lethargy, lack of motivation to achieve or exert effort • Requires frequent direction • Risky behaviors; alcohol abuse • Impulsive sex activity • Peer rejection • Driving accidents • Discipline problems; and family conflict • Anger; quickly fluctuating emotions • Difficulty with authority • Significant lags in academic performance • Poor self esteem; hopelessness
Adult	• Seems unusually disorganized • Poor concentration • Doesn't finish things • Procrastinates • Behaves impulsively • Unpredictable, rapid changes in emotional expressions • Low self-esteem (performance anxiety) • Alcohol or substance abuse • Antisocial behavior; arrests • Shorter employment duration • Greater distress and maladjustment on measures of psychological disorders • Poorer verbal and nonverbal working memory

> drowsy and unresponsive, or sleeping poorly due to over-reactivity and restlessness

> ► Experiencing feeding difficulties because of irregular appetites, "picky eating," poor sucking, or crying to an extent that interfered with nutritional intake

Some infants, later diagnosed with ADHD, show motor and attention deficits. European investigators emphasize the diagnostic value and importance of *motor deficits* in young children.[43]

One possible link between ADHD and depression may be explained by a finding that depressed mothers tend to foster inattention among their infants by terminating their child's play more abruptly and frequently.[44]

motor deficits — underdeveloped motor movements and coordination based on expectations by age

ADHD Presentation at Preschool Age

Normal three- and four-year-old children often have a pattern of inattention and overactivity that may or may not be related to ADHD. Although many children at age three appear to have all ADHD symptoms, they are difficult to distinguish from normal children with difficult temperaments.[45] However, children who are severely hyperactive at preschool age tend to have more learning, developmental, and behavior problems well into adolescence.

Severe hyperactivity in preschool may be one of the first significant signs of the disorder and lead practitioners to diagnose ADHD.[46]

Another indicator of ADHD relates to physical symptoms. One study found that children with ADHD had a much higher incidence of gastrointestinal, respiratory, and skin problems.[47] Additionally, both symptom degree and duration (six months to one year) are important diagnostic factors. At this age, clinicians may need to evaluate symptoms over a longer time period than that required by DSM-IV (TR) criteria to determine if children will outgrow the behaviors.

The limited data on preschool children suggests cautious diagnosis and careful follow-up with counseling, even though the bulk of evidence suggests that stimulant treatment can be helpful in many cases.[48–50]

Currently, large ongoing studies of preschoolers are evaluating diagnostic validity in the youngest age groups as well as treatment effects over time.

ADHD Presentation During Middle Childhood (ages 6 – 12)

Middle childhood is the most common time for children to exhibit strong signs of ADHD. Most children seen at mental health clinics are close to nine years old. During these years, children face new demands to fit in and meet school expectations of sitting still, following structure, and sharing one teacher's attention with perhaps 30 other students.

Most referrals for ADHD assessment occur during the first, second, and third grades because of poor performance and/or behavior problems.

ADHD behaviors may be exacerbated by the structured, rote nature of many school tasks (e.g., feeling that assigned tasks are too difficult, easy, or boring). This results in the child receiving

reinforcement — any consequence that increases the frequency of the preceding behavior

behavioral impulsivity — calling out in class, fidgeting, and repeatedly leaving one's seat or getting up "just to check something"

cognitive impulsivity — making frequent mistakes, being disorganized, and producing sloppy work

Hyperactivity, impulsivity, and inattention interfere with the child's ability to socialize with teachers and peers. Children with ADHD are usually unpopular with peers because they are unable to:

▶ *Wait in line*
▶ *Remember and follow rules*
▶ *Be a "good loser" at games*
▶ *Curb their quick tempers*
▶ *Show empathy and consideration for others*

In contrast, studies also indicate that hyperactive-impulsive children are sometimes very popular because of their attention-seeking and clowning style.[54]

little or inconsistent *reinforcement* for learning tasks requiring effort. A chronic lack of reinforcement for sustained effort may lead children to "give up" and be labeled as "lazy." Children diagnosed with ADHD during middle childhood often begin to experience a pattern of academic and social failure that leads to poor self-esteem and depression (e.g., feeling stupid and disliked by other children). This pattern typically stems from *behavioral impulsivity* and *cognitive impulsivity* as well as social skills deficits.

Others may perceive a cognitive impulsive style as symptomatic of a writing or spelling disability (which may be true); however, the patient with ADHD will demonstrate better performance after treatment.

Social skills problems are also very common at this age; those with ADHD typically lack the ability to perform the skills they've learned when required. Therefore, treatment in the natural environment rather than in the clinician's office may be more effective.

Although typically diagnosed with ADHD up to 10 times less often than boys, girls are more likely to escape diagnostic notice because they typically are less disruptive, impulsive, and aggressive, and more likely to be shy and anxious, especially in the classroom.[51] In adulthood, females have approximately the same referral rate as men and would have been classified as inattentive if diagnosed as children.[51-53]

Two critical determinations that impact treatment choices are:

▶ Do the problems stem from a learning disability?
▶ How pervasive are the symptoms; do they occur in more than one setting?

"ADHD-like" symptoms that present only in the school setting may indicate possible learning disability and/or challenges with the learning environment, which can impact treatment choices.

From the Patient's Perspective

The doctor thinks that I have ADHD. She asked me and my mom a whole lot of questions. She asked all about how much trouble I've been in. My teacher even had to fill out a paper. I was really embarrassed, but Mom says it will help me get better. The doctor wants me to start taking some pills for this; she says it will help my squirminess and make me pay attention better. Maybe I will be able to think better at school.

ADHD Presentation in Adolescence

As children reach adolescence, their overt hyperactivity may decrease and be replaced with feelings of inner restlessness.[55]

Distinguishing ADHD from other disorders may be difficult in adolescents because:

▶ They are at a developmental stage where the risk of depression and other psychiatric illnesses is greater, and there is a greater likelihood of accumulating more comorbid disorders as they get older.

▶ Overt behavioral problems that were easily recognized in younger children disappear with residual symptoms that are often unapparent to teachers and parents.

▶ More family problems and self-esteem issues become apparent.[55]

▶ Drug/alcohol experimentation is often present, which complicates ADHD recognition and treatment. Drug/alcohol use is a frequent comorbid condition with ADHD in adolescence, and ADHD may be an important risk factor for drug and alcohol abuse.

▶ An attention disorder may have begun earlier in life and may coexist with antisocial behaviors. The troublesome nature of antisocial behavior (as well as drug or alcohol abuse) in adolescents may lead clinicians to overlook a possible long history of ADHD preceding current turmoil.

▶ Physical impulsivity may decrease but poor attention as well as cognitive and verbal impulsivity frequently remain. Adolescents with residual ADHD symptoms typically perform tasks unevenly. For instance, they may burst with creativity for one class project, and then forget to do their homework in another.

Research has been unable to completely identify which ADHD children are likely to continue with symptoms or develop other behavior disorders.[57] About 70 percent of children diagnosed with ADHD show some signs of the disorder continuing into adolescence. Of that 70 percent, half of the group continues to show symptoms of a coexisting conduct disorder, and two-thirds experience a substance abuse disorder some time in their lives. Those adolescents who do not experience continuing signs of ADHD tend to function the same as their "normal" peers.[38]

According to some studies, about 25 percent of youths with ADHD drop out of high school.[38] Teachers of the last grade completed consistently rated those students as inferior to others in areas such as: completing tasks, working independently, getting along with others, and being punctual.

It is important to question the adolescent and obtain a comprehensive self-report of problem behaviors, moods, and family functioning. Rating scales will typically show the same general areas of dysfunction as in the younger child, but the specific symptom presentation will look different.

Clinically useful predictors for children with ADHD being at risk for a persistent disorder include familiarity, adversity, and psychiatric comorbidity.[56]

Because the classroom environment typically requires extended listening, organization, and rote memorization, those suffering from ADHD have significant problems in school. Adolescents with ADHD are more likely to quit school before graduation.

Dropout rates may reflect a lack of the specific skills necessary to perform in a school situation as well as the cumulative educational deficits incurred by these children throughout their schooling.

ADHD Presentation in Adulthood

As children with ADHD reach adulthood, behavioral impulsivity and hyperactivity decrease. Although the target symptoms of hyperactivity, inattention, and impulsivity are still reported by many patients, only one-third to one-half report levels high enough to cause impairment in daily functioning. Thus, even though adults no longer reach full criteria for ADHD, they may still suffer from significant levels of impairment, such as:

► Changing jobs frequently

► Having trouble paying attention to tedious or boring tasks

► Being easily distracted from important tasks by the slightest interruption or new stimuli

► Making impulsive decisions related to money, travel, jobs, or social plans

► Having more driving accidents, with more severe injuries and more damage, than their normal peers[58]

Adults with an extensive history of ADHD, who have experienced failure situations at school, home, and in peer relationships, find that working and separating from their family of origin allow lifestyle choices that may better suit their needs. For instance, individuals labeled as failures because they can't sit still and listen well may succeed as motivational speakers or salespersons.

As those with ADHD mature, they may generally learn coping or compensation skills and may be able to concentrate or curb impulses. Because this takes energy away from other areas, they may be rigid or easily frustrated. They will often marry a spouse who takes over a structuring, organizing role that helps them. However, this role may eventually lead to spousal conflict and marital distress, making marital and family problems an important focus of adult ADHD assessment.

One important change adults with ADHD experience is an increase in the salience of cognitive impairments, best described as *deficits in executive functioning.*[59] Typical symptoms of executive dysfunction include:

► Being disorganized

► Being forgetful (e.g., making lists, then forgetting to use them)

► Losing things

► Failing to plan ahead

► Depending on others for maintaining order

► Not being able to keep track of several things at once

► Not finishing projects or tasks

► Needing an absolute deadline in order to get things done

- ▶ Not being able to get started on tasks
- ▶ Changing plans/jobs in midstream
- ▶ Misjudging available time

While there appear to be important deficits in executive functioning in ADHD adults, it is important to remember that such deficits are not specific to ADHD and may be present in a number of other psychiatric disorders. Therefore, considering other possible disorders that can account for symptoms is important for diagnosis.[60-62]

Additionally, the risk for psychiatric disorders increases with age; thus, adults with ADHD are more likely than children to suffer from coexisting depression, anxiety, low self-esteem, and other psychiatric disorders. This makes differential diagnosis more difficult. Clinicians should consider these important symptoms of other disorders when making a diagnosis:

- ▶ Psychomotor agitation as well as diminished ability to think, concentrate, or make decisions (major depressive episode or dysthymia)
- ▶ Expansive or irritable mood, talkativeness, distractibility, excessive involvement in pleasurable activities with a high potential for painful consequences (manic or hypomanic episode)
- ▶ Trembling or shaking (panic disorder)
- ▶ Intrusive thoughts, repetitive behaviors, recurrent impulses, or restlessness arising from need to quell anxiety (obsessive-compulsive disorder)
- ▶ Difficulty concentrating, irritability, outbursts of anger, hypervigilance, exaggerated startle response (post-traumatic stress disorder)

What are the Specific DSM-IV (TR) Criteria for Diagnosing ADHD?

The **Diagnostic and Statistical Manual of Mental Disorders, Fourth Edition [DSM-IV(TR)]** outlines the criteria for establishing a diagnosis of ADHD and other mental disorders. DSM-IV(TR) addresses the debate over the role of hyperactivity, which historically had been a primary criterion, by including it as a subtype rather than a necessary or primary diagnostic component. DSM-IV(TR) organizes ADHD criteria into two subtypes:[1]

- ▶ Behavioral problems, such as hyperactivity and impulsivity
- ▶ Symptoms of inattention

Figure 2.3, on the following page, presents the current DSM-IV(TR) criteria for ADHD.

Though making a clinical ADHD diagnosis is complicated, long-term research studies, literature reviews, and medication responsiveness studies clearly substantiate the validity of ADHD as a mental disorder in adults.[37, 63, 64]

Appendix B covers ADHD differential diagnosis in detail.

The DSM-IV(TR), published in July 2000, altered the DSM-IV descriptive text based on empirical literature through 1992. It also corrected errors identified in the DSM-IV and changed diagnostic codes based on ICD-9-CM coding system updates. (ICD-9-CM is the coding system adopted by the U.S. Government and many foreign countries.

Figure 2.3   DSM-IV (TR) Criteria for Attention Deficit Hyperactivity Disorder

A. Either (1) or (2):

    (1) Six (or more) of the following symptoms of **inattention** have persisted for at least 6 months to a degree that is maladaptive and inconsistent with developmental level:

Inattention

    (a) often fails to give close attention to details or makes careless mistakes in schoolwork, work, or other activities

    (b) often has difficulty sustaining attention in tasks or play activities

    (c) often does not seem to listen when spoken to directly

    (d) often does not follow through on instructions and fails to finish schoolwork, chores, or duties in the workplace (not due to oppositional behavior or failure to understand instructions)

    (e) often has difficulty organizing tasks and activities

    (f) often avoids, dislikes, or is reluctant to engage in tasks that require sustained mental effort (such as schoolwork or homework)

    (g) often loses things necessary for tasks or activities (e.g., toys, school assignments, pencils, books, or tools)

    (h) is often easily distracted by extraneous stimuli

    (i) is often forgetful in daily activities

    (2) six (or more) of the following symptoms of **hyperactivity-impulsivity** have persisted for at least 6 months to a degree that is maladaptive and inconsistent with developmental level:

Hyperactivity

    (a) often fidgets with hands or feet or squirms in seat

    (b) often leaves seat in classroom or in other situations in which remaining seated is expected

    (c) often runs about or climbs excessively in situations in which it is inappropriate (in adolescents or adults, may be limited to subjective feelings of restlessness)

    (d) often has difficulty playing or engaging in leisure activities quietly

    (e) is often "on the go" or often acts as if "driven by a motor"

    (f) often talks excessively

Impulsivity

    (g) often blurts out answers before questions have been completed

    (h) often has difficulty awaiting turn

    (i) often interrupts or intrudes on others (e.g., butts into conversations or games)

B. Some hyperactive-impulsive or inattentive symptoms that caused impairment were present before age 7 years.

C. Some impairment from the symptoms is present in two or more settings (e.g., at school [or work] and at home).

D. There must be clear evidence of clinically significant impairment in social, academic, or occupational functioning.

E. Occurrence is not exclusively during the course of a Pervasive Developmental Disorder, Schizophrenia, or other Psychotic Disorder and is not better accounted for by another mental disorder (e.g., Mood Disorder, Anxiety Disorder, Dissociative Disorder, or a Personality Disorder).

Code based on type:

314.01   **Attention-Deficit/Hyperactivity Disorder, Combined Type:**
        if both Criteria A1 and A2 are met for the past 6 months

314.00   **Attention-Deficit/Hyperactivity Disorder, Predominantly Inattentive Type:**
        if Criterion A1 is met but Criterion A2 is not met for the past 6 months.

314.01   **Attention-Deficit/Hyperactivity Disorder, Predominantly Hyperactive-Impulsive Type:**
        if Criterion A2 is met but Criterion A1 is not met for the last 6 months.

Coding note: For individuals (especially adolescents and adults) who currently have symptoms that no longer meet full criteria, "In Partial Remission" should be specified.

(Reprinted with permission by the American Psychiatric Association: **Diagnostic and Statistical Manual of Mental Disorders, Fourth Edition, Text Revision,** Washington, DC, American Psychiatric Association, 1994)

Diagnostic Criteria for Adults with ADHD

Some authors argue that different criteria should be used when diagnosing adults versus children. As yet, there are no consensus guidelines for diagnosing ADHD among adults. One prominent authority suggests criteria that include:[65]

- Persistent motor activity
- Attention deficits, including:
  - Inability to keep mind on conversation
  - Distractibility
  - Inability to concentrate on reading materials
  - Difficulty focusing on the job
  - Frequent forgetfulness
- *Affective lability*
- Inability to complete tasks
- Hot temper
- Impulsivity
- Low tolerance for stress

affective lability — marked and rapid mood shifts

Other authors suggest that, in addition to a childhood history of ADD and symptoms not explained by another medical or psychiatric condition, one of the following criteria is needed for the diagnosis:[66]

- Sense of underachievement
- Difficulty getting organized
- Chronic procrastination
- Trouble with following through
- Blurting out what comes to mind
- Search for high levels of stimulation
- Intolerance of boredom
- Easy distractibility; "tuning out"
- Often creative, highly intelligent, flashes of brilliance
- Trouble following established procedures
- Impatience and low tolerance for frustration
- Impulsivity, either verbally or in action
- Tendency to worry needlessly
- Sense of insecurity
- Mood swings; mood lability
- Restlessness
- Tendency to addictive behavior
- Chronic problems with self-esteem
- Inaccurate self-observation
- Family history of ADD, manic-depressive illness, depression, or substance abuse

These very broad symptom criteria may open the door to several other disorders and have not been empirically verified in controlled studies.

When these symptoms are included in rating scales that also include childhood symptoms, they resolve into only four major clusters:[67]

1. Inattention/Cognitive Problems
2. Hyperactivity/Restlessness
3. Impulsivity/Emotional Lability
4. Problems with Self-Concept

Adult ADHD appears to reflect the same basic dimensions found in childhood rating scale analyses.

Many of the symptoms described by others as problems in executive functioning (such as procrastination, failure to complete tasks, poor organization and planning, poor memory) fall into a broad category of inattention and cognitive problems. These results tend to confirm similar clusters of symptoms to those found for ADHD in children, with the addition of low self-concept and self-esteem.[67]

Additional Clarifying Information for Diagnosing Children and Adults

Simply knowing that typical ADHD symptoms are present is not enough for a rigorous and accurate diagnosis. The most common ADHD diagnostic mistake is to rely only on symptoms. Most normal people have some symptoms some of the time; many other disorders have some or all of the ADHD symptoms. Clinicians should note the following about these symptoms:

There are many other mental and medical disorders that present symptoms of inattention or hyperactivity, including acute infections, post-traumatic stress, and substance intoxication or withdrawal. In these cases, the prominent mental or medical condition is diagnosed while treatment for the ADHD symptoms may still take place. For example, a child with severe mental retardation, who also meets all of the ADHD criteria, may respond well to stimulant medication yet remain severely impaired and represent a separate diagnostic entity from more-typical ADHD.[68]

▶ **Age of onset of the disorder** — Only some symptoms must occur before age seven, but these must be severe enough to create impairment. For example, the clinician may establish that some hyperactive-impulsive symptoms were present in kindergarten, but if those symptoms created no impairment in social, academic, or home functioning, the age-of-onset criterion would not be met. However, over 40 percent of children with the inattentive subtype failed to meet the age-seven onset criterion, so flexibility regarding this criterion is important.

▶ **Number and severity of symptoms** — DSM-IV requires the presence of at least six of nine hyperactive-impulsive symptoms, and/or six of nine inattentive symptoms. However, these symptoms must occur **often** and they must be "maladaptive and inconsistent with developmental level." The clinician must determine the symptom severity with reference to developmental and normative expectations at a given age.

▶ **Pervasiveness and severity of impairment —** Impairment must occur in two or more settings (e.g., social, academic, or occupational) and there must be evidence that the degree of impairment is "clinically significant." Like symptom severity, clinical significance varies with developmental expectations for age and gender.

▶ **Persistence** — The symptoms must have persisted for at least six months with no sustained or intermittent lapses. Symptoms of excitability or inattention could be due to a recent trauma, onset of depression, substance abuse, or organic disease. These symptoms would not count towards ADHD symptom criteria because they did not persist over a six-month period.

▶ **Alternative diagnoses and coexisting mental disorders** — ADHD symptoms cannot be present only during the course of another disorder, for example: pervasive developmental disorder, schizophrenia, an anxiety disorder, or a depressive disorder. See appendix B for more information on differentiating ADHD from other disorders.

What Assessment Techniques Can Be Used to Diagnose ADHD?

Since there are no definitive ADHD diagnostic tests that clearly demarcate "normal" behaviors from ADHD symptoms, clinicians use a combination of interview, observation, and standardized assessment measurements to assess ADHD symptoms, impairment, and differential diagnoses.[69]

Interview and History Techniques

Family, psychiatric, developmental, and medical histories as well as patient and parent interviews are the most important methods of assessing the history and symptom picture for ADHD in children and adults. Clinicians need to gather a complete social, medical, and developmental history (from conception to present) to differentiate between situational problems, other diagnoses, and ADHD. This information also affects treatment planning.

Although it is relatively easy to identify the presence of ADHD symptoms, clinicians find it more difficult to determine whether those symptoms seem excessive for the patient's developmental stage and whether the symptoms are chronic and pervasive enough to warrant an ADHD diagnosis. As a result, clinicians use careful interviewing while also comparing symptoms to normative behavioral standards for the patient's age and gender, based upon rating scales.

Thorough interview techniques determine whether the patient's behavior differs significantly from "normal" peers. For example, a child who has "difficulty following through on instructions from others" may do so only:

▶ *In certain situations (school, doing chores)*

▶ *With certain individuals (parents or employers)*

▶ *When instructions are complex*

Clinicians often ask parents and teachers to complete standardized rating scales before the interview itself. The interviewer then focuses on those symptoms rated as "often" or "very often" on the rating scales.[70]

Assessing ADHD in adults places more emphasis on self-report techniques. Also, observations by the patient's significant others (e.g., spouse, sibling, roommate, employer) become crucial as adult ADHD patients often lack significant insight into their own behavior.

Personal areas (e.g., participation in sports, hobbies, music, or recreational activities) illuminate the patient's functioning as a result of their symptoms. Conceptualized as broad, "quality-of-life" issues, personal functioning may be impaired in those of all ages with ADHD.[71]

Other areas to assess for specific home, school, peer, and self impairments include:

► *Paying attention to detail*
► *Sustaining attention*
► *Listening*
► *Finishing tasks*
► *Organizing*
► *Sustaining effort*
► *Keeping track of things*
► *Being distracted*
► *Being forgetful*
► *Fidgeting or squirming*
► *Leaving seat*
► *Playing quietly*
► *Appearing to be driven, on the go*
► *Talking excessively*
► *Blurting out*
► *Interrupting*

Appendix A provides a list of commonly used teacher rating scales.

To assess impairment, clinicians explore ADHD symptoms in at least four main areas or domains of functioning:

► School or job performance
► Family and home environment
► Social relationships
► Personal functioning (self), including: self-image, belief in one's abilities, and mood

When interviewing, ask for specific examples of each characteristic and its impact on daily functioning. The 18-item DSM-IV symptom list can serve as an interview guide for probing areas of functioning. For example, if the parent agrees that the child, "Does not seem to listen . . . ," then the clinician may ask how that affects:

► Schoolwork or job performance
► Ability to interact with peers or co-workers
► Playing sports
► Following directions at home or on the job

Specific examples, articulated in the patient's own words, help determine the effects of ADHD on functioning. These examples are also the basis for evaluating change due to treatment interventions. After treatment begins, one can monitor how the treatment affects hyperactivity, impulsivity, or inattention. Figure 2.4, on the next page, provides examples of one child's symptom descriptions for home, school, social, and self domains of functioning.

To qualify for an ADHD diagnosis, a significant level of impairment from symptoms must be present. In many ways, impairment is the actual target of interventions, since many people have symptoms without corresponding impairment.[72]

School or Job Performance

In assessing school performance in children, the fact that children frequently minimize the severity or significance of their difficulties makes parent and teacher input essential for diagnosis. Listed below are a number of validated tools and techniques for assessing school-related aspects of ADHD:

► **Teacher rating scales** — These are usually the most efficient way to provide critical information. During an initial assessment, such scales should cover at least one month of the child's functioning with a particular classroom teacher. In follow-up assessments, shorter periods with more targeted scales may be used in assessing changes due to treatment interventions.[73, 74]

► **Observable behaviors at school** — Teachers can often identify children with ADHD through specific

Figure 2.4   Diagnostic Interview Notes:
Assessing ADHD Target Symptoms and Domains of Impairment

DSM-IV Symptom	Home	School or Job	Peers	Self
...makes careless mistakes	Mom says he doesn't check his homework and is constantly missing problems that she knows he knows how to do	Skips items on tests; doesn't check his assignments before handing them in	Always messes up in team sports, so gets ridiculed by peers	Says he is dumb at school
...doesn't seem to listen	Mom has to repeat things several times before he does a chore (but he is not oppositional about it)	Doesn't write down assignments that teacher gives orally; teacher wonders if he has a hearing problem	Has to be reminded when playing soccer and baseball where he is supposed to stand to play his position	Says people are always mad at him because he doesn't seem to hear when spoken to
...often runs about	Wakes everybody up early by his running noisily all over the house	Up and out of seat without cause and without permission; teacher gives many reprimands	Friends call him "hyper" and "retard" because he won't sit still in board games	Says he must be stupid as kids call him names, and he does poorly on school work
...difficulty waiting turn in line	Jumps his turn when playing video game with brother	Runs to head of the line and gets reprimanded	Friends pick him last for games because he is always going out of turn	Says he feels sad because kids don't like the way he acts

behaviors, such as students who talk to themselves, talk out loud without permission, get out of their seat without permission, or fail to have appropriate materials (e.g., pencil or eraser). One study found these combined variables predicted teacher ratings of ADHD in 83 percent of cases, though there was considerable overlap with non-ADHD students.[75]

▶ **Grades and report cards** — These provide significant ADHD-related indicators. Look for comments about impulsiveness, disruptive behavior, or attendance. These indicators help determine if poor grades stem from ADHD or actual skill deficits.

▶ **Homework assignments** — These frequently allow parents to clearly observe a child's work habits and skills deficits. Changes in homework completion can also indicate response to treatment.

▶ **The amount of frustration, stress, and struggle related to school or homework** — These often indicate a child's inability to stay on task, work independently, and self-correct mistakes. However, the clinician must determine whether these signs reflect an attention deficit, a learning disability, or teaching materials poorly suited to the child's ability.

Figure 2.5   ADHD Severity Rating Guidelines[78]

Standards for measuring impairment are generally quite loose and informal. One well-developed measure, the Child and Adolescent Functional Assessment Scale, is available, but is usually too long and complex for most clinical situations.[76] A relatively brief overall impairment scale is also available.[77]

Using clinical practice experience, the guidelines on these two pages provide an estimate of severity of impairment.[78]

Instructions	*The following categories for rating the severity of illness are meant to provide **general guidelines**. The suggested examples are not exhaustive. Some patients will have symptoms or aspects of functioning that do not appear in the list. Some may have behaviors or characteristics that fit into more than one category. Clinicians should nevertheless try to make their best estimate as to the level of functioning based on the closest overall match to the categories.*
Normal, no impairment	• Personal distress is minimal and is no more than experienced by the average person of this age and personal situation. Ups and downs occur but are experienced as a normal part of life and do not impair accomplishment of major goals. • Able to attend, focus on tasks, complete assignments or manage normal routines, remember things, and use good judgement. Self-esteem is high. • Able to set goals and accomplish them. • Is no more scattered or forgetful than is appropriate for age. • Functions well in job; or if student, functions as well as can be expected given his/her aptitude and background . • Functions very well interpersonally and in family interactions. Controls impulses to talk out of turn. Few lapses in judgement with a consistent level of self-control. Doesn't tread on others' toes. Calm and attentive to others' needs. • Family and friends regard him/her as basically a normal person who functions extremely well in just about all areas of life related to ADHD.
Borderline impairment	• Occasional difficulty focusing on tasks, but generally able to do well with little extra effort. • Has some forgetfulness, such as misplacing keys or work materials; but basically this is a nuisance rather than any real impairment of work, study, or social obligation. • Experiences some mild difficulty in sitting through lectures, concerts, or social gatherings, but most people would be unaware of this; he/she is able to function quite well to all appearances and does not appear as notably restless. • Occasional lapses of judgement in saying inappropriate things or in decisions, but on the whole maintains a pretty consistent level of self-control. • Family members or close acquaintances find him/her to be mildly quirky, fidgety, impulsive in speech or action; but mostly they see a normal person who has occasional lapses that they do not take too seriously.

Mild Impairment	• Has some impairment in a single area of functioning (work/school, home, social/interpersonal, self-esteem). • The level of impairment due to ADHD is such that it causes a definite problem needing some treatment, but it does not cause a serious breakdown, such as threatening one's job, marriage, ability to finish school, ability to make and keep friends, etc. Would like treatment but does not feel it absolutely necessary. • Persistent inability to accomplish all that he or she wants, but on the whole is able to do most of what is desired by applying extra effort. • Some areas of limitation in fulfilling ones abilities to the fullest. • Others tend to view this person as having some problems.
Moderate impairment	• Has some impairment in at least two areas of functioning (work/school, home, social/interpersonal, self-esteem). • The level of impairment is significant but not extreme. There is some threat to job level or security; or to good relations with family or friends, or to continued academic functioning; but things are not yet at a critical stage.
Marked impairment	• There is impairment due to ADHD in three or more areas of life (work/school, home, social/interpersonal, self-esteem) to a substantial degree. • The level of impairment is such that there is a likely threat to continued functioning, such as loss of job, dropping out of school, breakup of marriage, or a significant loss of friends or supporters. • He or she may already have gotten into serious difficulties because of their restlessness, impulsive behavior, stimulus seeking, or disregard for socially appropriate behavior. • Chronically unable to manage responsibilities (home care, managing money, child care, chores, appointments, etc.); always into trouble for inability to start or finish tasks.
Severe Impairment	• There is some impairment in virtually all four areas of life (work/school, home, social/interpersonal, self-esteem). • There is a substantial interference of functioning in one or more areas which causes great difficulty in sustaining a marriage, holding a job, or staying in school. • Significant treatment is required or further erosion of areas of functioning will likely occur. • Severely impaired and unable without assistance or treatment, to change behavior to meet responsibilities, etc.
Maximal, profound impairment	• Severe difficulties in most areas of life (e.g., can't hold a job, has no friends due to impulsive behavior, unable to have a close relationship, can't concentrate on school tasks or sit still long enough to enjoy leisure). • Most areas of functioning severely affected because of impulsivity, restlessness, or inability to concentrate.

Educational and/or psychological testing can clarify how learning disorders impair school performance and differentiate these learning disorders from ADHD.

▶ **A poor fit between the child's capabilities and the level of instruction** — This is the most common reason for poor school work.[79] Research demonstrates that inattentiveness negatively affects reading achievement as well as attitudes about reading. But findings also indicate strong reciprocal effects; that is, reading achievement affects attentiveness in the classroom. Therefore, someone who is a poor reader could have a learning disability in reading and display poor attention because of frustrations, or could be a poor reader because of concentration difficulties due to ADHD.[80]

▶ **Messiness of the child's desk at school** — This is a good indicator of organization and attention to rules.[75]

▶ **Poor peer relationships at school** — These often reflect poor social skills due to problems obeying rules (impulsivity) during play activities.

Assessing job performance in adults can be difficult as adults can be poor reporters of their behavior at home and at work. Therefore, whenever possible, include a significant other (e.g., spouse, roommate, girl friend, etc.) in the adult patient assessment. The history of working adults or college students with ADHD often reveal that adult patients:

Many young adults with ADHD in school or college suffered similar school-related difficulties as children.

▶ **Change jobs or colleges frequently** — Often an adult with ADHD changes jobs frequently due to "boredom" or inability to complete routine tasks. Many employers also terminate employment when the individual fails to cope with task demands, to be punctual, or to sustain the ability to work towards goals. College students may drop out frequently and have difficulty with studying, homework, and completing assignments on time.

▶ **Procrastinate** — Missed deadlines and difficulty completing tasks or ideas often dominate the work history of adult patients with ADHD. They frequently admit that they complete tasks only under threat of severe consequences. For example, an artist complains that he never finishes portraits in the time commissioned. Or, a computer analyst writes brilliant code, but produces a report only after being threatened with a salary cut.

▶ **Have interpersonal difficulties and poor social skills** — Interpersonal difficulties are often noted by supervisors and coworkers and typically include "foot-in-the-mouth" statements reflecting impulsive verbal traits.

▶ **Exhibit extreme fluctuations in behavior** — These fluctuations characterize many with ADHD. Sometimes, they show creativity or bursts of energy in completing certain tasks; often ADHD patients have difficulty being creative or energetic consistently.

Family and Individual Psychiatric Histories

Family and individual psychiatric histories help in making an accurate diagnosis. Specifically, family-genetic studies show a significant likelihood of several psychiatric conditions in first-degree relatives (i.e., mother, father, and siblings) of children with ADHD.[81-84] These include:

- ADHD
- Affective and anxiety disorders
- Learning disorders
- Conduct, oppositional, and antisocial disorders
- Alcohol and substance abuse
- Antisocial personality disorders

Family history may provide clues to diagnosis. For instance, someone whose parents have both been diagnosed with ADHD will be more likely to be diagnosed with ADHD. Children with a parent having bipolar disorder are at higher risk for bipolar disorder. The related symptoms, such as irritable mood, talkativeness, racing thoughts, distractibility, and impulsive behavior, may be easily confused with ADHD.

> *Often the only clue as to the meaning of symptoms in a patient being assessed for ADHD is the genetically loaded family history.*

Similarly, children with a family history of affective disorders, or who were diagnosed with affective disorders in childhood, show many behaviors that might be misinterpreted as ADHD.[85, 86] Some symptoms (e.g., loss of interest or pleasure, psychomotor agitation, poor concentration, and feelings of worthlessness) often reflect a depressive mood disorder that can be mistaken for ADHD. Likewise, symptoms due to post-traumatic stress disorder (PTSD) may be misinterpreted as ADHD symptoms. A child's symptoms may relate, in part, to a chronically chaotic home life due to marital conflict, alcohol abuse, physical or sexual abuse, or psychiatric illness of a family member. Of course, such conditions may be present along with true ADHD and may affect the outcome of the disorder.

Psychiatric histories of both the patient and the family should include an assessment of:

- Depression
- Mania
- Anxiety
- Thought or perceptual disturbances

> *Mental disorders with symptoms similar to ADHD include bipolar disorder, conduct disorder, affective disorders, depressive mood disorder, learning disabilities, anxiety disorders, and borderline personality disorder. See appendix B for differential diagnostic information.*

This assessment helps determine what diagnoses may be differential versus coexisting and whether or not there are symptoms of a single disorder or multiple disorders at the same time.

Medical and Developmental History

Clinicians should gather a thorough medical and developmental history to identify causal factors that may stem from certain medical conditions as well as to establish any pattern of ADHD *maladaptive behavior.* From a medical standpoint, there are several risk factors associated with ADHD that should be noted by the clinician. These include:

maladaptive behavior — behavior that leads to excessive distress, typically requiring therapy

> ► Prenatal and postnatal difficulties, such as toxemia, trauma, infection during pregnancy, or the baby having difficulty breathing, sucking, or sleeping shortly after birth.

> ► Maternal substance abuse, particularly alcohol and cigarettes during pregnancy.

> ► Poor maternal health.

Certain physical disorders can have symptoms similar to ADHD. For more information, see appendix B.

> ► Vitamin/mineral deficiencies can simulate ADHD symptoms, though foods do not cause ADHD. Sub-clinical vitamin deficiencies can cause inattention and lowered test performance.[87] Lead and cadmium can be absorbed into the brain, causing hyperactivity and learning disabilities. [88-90]

Children with certain medical conditions, such as hyperthyroidism, seizures, hearing problems, allergies (e.g., corn, peanuts, or milk), or various genetic disorders, can have symptoms that mimic ADHD symptoms. Another common problem is the confusion between children's inattention to verbal stimuli and their hearing acuity.[91]

Despite research results to the contrary, many people continue to believe that sugar intake causes hyperactivity or mood changes in children.

From a developmental standpoint, parents often report signs of hyperactivity before birth (especially in the third trimester). As babies, these children reach developmental milestones, such as walking, talking, or interactive play, in an erratic fashion. Some skills may be acquired early; others are delayed. For example, parents may report that their child "went from a crawl to a run" when starting to walk but did not speak in full sentences until much later than siblings. ADHD children may sleep less and quit taking naps early. Parents find them difficult to manage as they constantly move from one activity to the next and may report that their toys never last because of vigorous play and accidents.

Medical histories often reveal associations between certain medical factors and ADHD, including:

> ► *Multiple ear infections that may interfere with spatial localization of speech sounds and with attention to speech[92]*

> ► *Headaches*

> ► *Frequent illnesses*

> ► *Poor hand-eye coordination*

> ► *Left-handedness (not directly associated with ADHD, but more common in children with ADHD whose parents have depressive illness[37])*

> ► *Being accident prone*

Utilizing a Specific Interview Format

In research studies and clinical practice, formal instruments are often used to document the ADHD diagnosis and rule out alternative diagnoses. Their reliability and validity have been extensively studied, and they provide acceptable documentation for managing care and compiling data for clinical research. The most commonly used structured interviews include:

> ► NIMH Diagnostic Interview Schedule for Children (DISC)[93]

> ► Diagnostic Interview for Children and Adolescents (DICA)[94]

> ► Schedule for Affective Disorders and Schizophrenia for School-Age Children (Kiddie-SADS)[95]
>
> ► Conners Adult ADHD Diagnostic Interview for DSM-IV[96]

Brief forms for development, medical history, treatment history, and social history have been developed for child and adult ADHD.[97] A brief structured interview, targeting ADHD and oppositional/conduct problems, is also available.[98]

Clinical Interviewing of the Adult

Adult interview techniques target retrospective and current symptoms. Some of the DSM-IV(TR) criteria clearly designate some symptoms as adult, such as "careless mistakes in . . . work" or "subjective feelings of restlessness." However, most of the diagnostic criteria relate to children because some symptoms must be present before the age of seven. Some researchers advocate relaxing this age criterion where adult patients are concerned.[100]

An often-used interview technique involves asking an adult to recall childhood behaviors. Verifying early ADHD symptoms in an adult is difficult since retrospective childhood histories may be erroneous. Because contact with an adult's family members is often impossible, asking for and interpreting historical information requires extreme care. However, some evidence shows that using the Wender Utah Rating Scale (reviewed in appendix A) provides valid recall. Adult patients are asked to fill this out retrospectively, ". . . as I was as a child."[65, 101] Norms have been developed for adult recall of the 18 DSM-IV(TR) symptoms in childhood as well as for current adult functioning.[100]

Another interview format uses the 18 DSM symptoms, asking the patient to rate them on a four-point scale of severity.[38, 102] Since overt, observable symptoms are often not as prominent in adulthood, subtler interview questions may reveal pertinent information. For example, clinicians should ask questions about whether it "feels" hard to sit still, rather than asking about "squirming." They should ask if an adult patient seems to have more energy than others do, rather than asking about excessive energy.

Cognitions or thinking patterns may reflect inattention or impulsivity. For example, information about whether adult patients see themselves as detail-oriented or organized can be important. This can be verified by asking about the status of their checkbook, neatness of their home or desk at work, or for the plot of a book, movie, or TV show they recently experienced. The amount of time spent in these activities is also a clue.

Decision-making and social interactions can also demonstrate impulsivity. Ask the patient questions such as:

> ► Do you take time to make decisions or jump into change?
>
> ► Are you an impulse buyer?

For more information on these assessment measures, see appendix A.

ADHD is the most common psychiatric condition among children with speech and language disorders and is often associated with verbal learning disabilities.[99]

Many studies indicate poor recollection of past events, moods, and behaviors, especially when evaluating the degree of intensity. Some evidence indicates that the patient's parents have more accurate recall than the adult patient.

When asking questions about employment, ask what specific tasks patients enjoy and which they avoid. For example, they may avoid paperwork or accounting, while starting new projects may be a favorite activity. In addition, ask patients to rate the amount of attention needed in their work, and what type of job they would like if they could improve their concentration.

Common complaints and observations in adults with ADHD include:[103]

▶ *Rapid, brief mood shifts or over-excitability*
▶ *Constant purposeless motion of extremities*
▶ *Hot temper*
▶ *Distractibility*
▶ *Low self-esteem; feeling of inadequacy*
▶ *Disinhibitions*
▶ *Stress intolerance; feeling chronically overwhelmed*
▶ *Disorganization in answering open-ended questions*
▶ *Disorganization and inefficiency*
▶ *Poor ability to follow long explanations*
▶ *Procrastinates without absolute deadlines*
▶ *Obsessive-compulsive, stimulus-seeking, or antisocial behaviors*
▶ *Inability to relax*
▶ *Stubbornness*
▶ *Restless sleep*
▶ *Excessively active lifestyle*
▶ *Forgetfulness*
▶ *Failure to plan ahead*
▶ *Inability to multitask*
▶ *Failure to judge task durations*
▶ *Inability to complete tasks*
▶ *Speaking or making decisions without considering consequences*
▶ *Failure to live up to occupational potential*
▶ *Difficulty keeping jobs or sustaining relationships*
▶ *Family violence*
▶ *Alcohol or other drug (especially caffeine) abuse*
▶ *Driving Problems (accidents, traffic violations)*

▶ Do you make decisions on the spot in response to sudden, strong emotions?

▶ Are you easily frustrated or angered?

Patients may report feelings of restlessness or irritability when subjected to quiet or sedentary activities, but may not show actual signs of excessive movement. Information regarding frequency, intensity, and coping methods helps indicate the extent of the problem.

A significant problem in assessing adults by interview (and to a lesser extent when assessing children through parental report) is an individual who exaggerates symptoms in order to obtain services or get a prescription for a stimulant medication. The only real safeguard against sophisticated patients who have memorized symptom criteria or who have read enough popular accounts of ADHD to fool the unwary interviewer is a thorough developmental interview. Such an interview assesses the total pattern of findings, including level of impairment, that leads to accurate ADHD diagnosis.

Observation Techniques

Direct patient observation is critical to ADHD diagnosis. Though seldom an option, observing patients in a natural setting, (e.g., classroom, seminar or meeting, work setting) can greatly enhance diagnosis. However, clinicians can assess overactivity, inattention, impulsivity, and compliance with instructions in their own office, keeping in mind the situation's uniqueness and the fact that the clinician's one-on-one attention may suppress typical behaviors, especially in children. Adults, on the other hand, manifest most problems in their behavioral style. These may include inability to focus, inability to organize a chronological account of their problems, sensitivity to social rejection, tardiness, and inaccuracies in filling out forms.

Begin observing patients from the moment they enter the waiting room, office, or any other setting. Comments such as, "I had a hard time finding this place," may reflect chronic difficulties in map-reading or spatial memory, or just inattention to cues. In the office, pay attention to signs of:

▶ **Motor restlessness** — Do patients fidget, tap their fingers or feet, or explore the room?

▶ **Attention and impulsivity** — What are patients' responses to being asked to wait, asked long and "boring" questions, or filling out forms and questionnaires?

▶ **Social and relational skills** — How do patients interact with significant others who accompany them, and how do they relate to the clinician or examiner? (This is especially important with adults, since other types of observation may be impractical.)

Observing Children

Structured observation with children allows the clinician to compare symptoms with same-aged peers and note situational variables (e.g., what tasks the child performs and the type and frequency of reinforcement they receive).

One method of structured observation for children involves recording several classroom behaviors, such as being out of the seat, straying off-task, or talking out of turn during 15- or 30-second intervals. Observation periods may alternate between the child and one or more same-sex peers. This method allows direct symptom comparison with a "normal" peer group for diagnosis or ongoing evaluation of behavior changes due to treatment. The key behaviors most often associated with ADHD in the classroom are off-task behaviors, gross-motor movements, and interference with others. Detailed behavioral definitions of these and other target behaviors are available in published coding systems.[104] Another observation method is the Child Behavior Checklist-Direct Observation Form (CBCL-DOF).[105]

Some research indicates that a teacher's global estimate of time on task is reasonably reliable, correlates moderately well with direct observations, and does not require specially trained observers.

Although structured observation techniques seem promising, reports conflict as to how well the results correlate with ratings obtained from parents and/or teachers. Direct observations are apparently more valid because they represent carefully defined samples of behavior taken directly. However, the high cost of training to use this method and the limited time for clinicians to visit the classroom may make this approach unfeasible. Additionally, these small pictures of behavior may not take into account the appropriateness or relevance to the setting usually supplied in more global observations by teachers. Nevertheless, a recent review of several studies using observation concluded that these techniques are valuable when used in a structured manner in conjunction with other methods.[106]

Some schools require informed consent to observe a child in the classroom. Pediatricians or other physicians may be able to enlist the services of the school psychologist for making in-class observations during an assessment. For evaluation purposes, school psychologists may be able to visit the classroom for observations without special permission.

Observing Adolescents

Clinicians use observation less with adolescents than with children. Peer relations are very important for those in this age group, and observation may be *stigmatizing*. Adolescents are typically more aware of the observation, and *reactivity effects* may increase at this age. In addition, the differences in an adolescent's environment may make direct observation more difficult. For example, classes are shorter, there are numerous classrooms and teachers, and some classes require more movement (e.g., woodworking or physical education).

stigmatizing — a mark on one's reputation

reactivity effects — different behaviors than usual, caused by being watched

Observing Adults

Clinicians have generally ignored observation techniques in assessments of adults. This is due, in part, to the reduction of overt signs of inattention and hyperactivity that occur as an individual matures. In addition, problems can arise when a clinician attempts to unobtrusively watch someone in the workplace. For example, observation may cause disruption of work flow, lead to embarrassment or questions from coworkers, or possibly jeopardize a patient's work status. However, it may be possible to observe and compare behavior during seminars, meetings, or college classes.

Standardized Assessment Measures

Various behavior rating scales can be used to assess ADHD. These scales are easy to administer, can be completed quickly, and quantify how behavior deviates from norms for a particular age and gender. Questionnaires elicit parent and teacher observations, while self-reports provide valuable information from children, adolescents, and adults. Besides helping with initial diagnosis, these tools can aid clinicians in conducting follow-up assessments of treatment efficacy.

Appendix A provides complete descriptions of the specific instruments listed in this section.

The following overview explains various assessment measures currently in use. Appendix A provides more detailed information on each of these measures. Comprehensive handbooks are available with a complete description of these tools.[107, 108] Types of instruments available are:

- ► **Clinician observation tool** — The CBCL-Direct Observation Form is a structured observation measure that helps assess a broad spectrum of symptoms.[105]

- ► **Parent ratings** — The most commonly used parent rating measures are the Conners Parent Rating Scales (CPRS) and the Child Behavior Check List (CBCL).[105] The Conners Scales (teacher, parent, adolescent self-report, and adult) have been newly *standardized* on a large, national sample. Less commonly used parent rating scales are the ADHD Rating Scale and the Home Situations Questionnaire-Revised (HSQ-R).[109]

standardized — data collected on a large group and results put in the form of averages by age group and gender

- ► **Teacher ratings** — To validate an ADHD diagnosis, the clinician should obtain ratings from adults besides parents who observe the child's behavior in different settings. The most common questionnaires available assess teachers' observations. These include:
  - ■ Conners Teacher Rating Scales — Revised (CTRS-R)[110]
  - ■ Child Behavior Checklist — Teacher's Report Form (CBCL-TRF)[105]

Commonly used self-rating scales are:

- ► *Child Behavior Check List-Youth Self Report Form (CBCL-YSR)*
- ► *Wender Utah Rating Scale (Adult)*
- ► *Conners/Wells Adolescent Self-Report of Symptoms (CASS)*
- ► *Conners Adult Attention-Deficit Rating Scale (CAARS)*

- ► **Self ratings (child and adult)** — Common self report forms include:
  - ■ CBCL's Youth Self-Report form (CBCL-YSR)[111]
  - ■ Wender Utah Rating Scale (WURS).[65]
  - ■ An adolescent, self-report scale (CASS) that has been standardized on over 6,000 children from 12 to 18 years[110]
  - ■ An adult, self- and significant-other scale (CAARS)[112]

▶ **Neuropsychological tests** — With increased acceptance of the theory that ADHD involves impairment
of frontal lobe functioning, use of neuropsychological
testing for diagnosis has become more popular. Several
research studies use these objective measures for
assessment.[113] However, neuropsychological testing is
better for determining the absence of ADHD than it is
for verifying the diagnosis. Poor performance on these
tests can either result from symptoms of ADHD or a
variety of extraneous factors. For example, motivation
and reinforcement for performance can be affected by
the structure and novelty of the testing situation and
the clinician's one-on-one attention. Depression, learning disabilities, or anxiety are other possible causes of
impaired scores. Commonly used neuropsychological
tests (reviewed in detail in appendix A) include:

■ Continuous Performance Test (CPT)[114]

■ Freedom From Distractibility Factor (FD) on the
WISC and WAIS intelligence scales[115]

■ Matching Familiar Figures Test (MFFT)[116]

■ Stroop Word-Color Association Test[117]

■ Wisconsin Card Sort[118]

■ Test of Working Memory[119]

▶ **Family functioning tests** — Clinicians should investi-
gate family situational factors to determine areas where
intervention may decrease problem behaviors. This
requires taking a psychosocial history that includes the
status of marital, parent/child, and sibling relationships
as well as communication styles. Family members
(including a child who has been diagnosed with ADHD)
generally exhibit a higher level of discord and pathology.
For example, one study found that long, parent-child
separations occur often in families with an ADHD child.
These separations negatively influence the outcome of
the disorder.[121] Clinicians should assess these factors
informally through an interview or by using standardized
tests that measure the family environment or parenting
stress, such as:

■ The Family Environment Scale[122, 123]

■ The Family Assessment Device[124]

■ The Parenting Stress Index[125]

All tests are best used to support interview and observation
results. Carefully choose a few measures to clarify diagnosis and
guide treatment planning.

*Neuropsychological testing
generally focuses on sustained
attention, impulsivity, and
neuropsychological or frontal
lobe functions.*

*Even though current research
has failed to demonstrate the
value of using these measures
with adult populations,
valuable observations about
behavioral style, impulse control,
reactivity, and attention can
be made when administering
structured cognitive tasks,
such as the Wechsler Adult
Intelligence Scales (WAIS) or
the Continuous Performance
Test (CPT). There is an audio
tape guide for using the CPT
as a source of behavioral
observations.[120]*

*Although not directly related
to the diagnosis of ADHD,
consideration of family
functioning is an important
part of the assessment and
helps in treatment planning.*

*For example, parent and
teacher questionnaires (such as
the CBCL or CTRS reviewed in
appendix A) are quick, reliable,
and can provide information for
follow-up during the interview.*

The level of family adversity significantly impacts ADHD. Low socioeconomic status (SES), large family size, parental criminal actions, and maternal mental disorder are related to greater ADHD impairment, including a decrease in intellectual ability.

Other measures can be selected according to specific needs. For example:

> ▶ Neuropsychological tests may be helpful after an interview indicating a history of neurological problems or learning disabilities. It is standard practice to obtain a measure of IQ and achievement in cases with suspected learning disabilities.

> ▶ A clinician may want to measure depression in patients having a family history of depression.

Assessing Changes Due to Treatment

multi-method approach — a treatment approach that uses observer ratings, interview, and testing both in clinical medication trials and in individual patient treatment

An important principle of evaluating the effects of treatment is a *multi-method approach*, which uses three steps to evaluate the effects of treatment:

1. Establishing target symptoms
2. Measuring domains of impairment
3. Measuring changes at different treatment intensities (e.g., medication dosage)

Establishing target symptoms — Therapies may address many possible target symptoms assessed by gathering information from teachers, parents, and directly from the child. To evaluate the impact of therapy, assess the specific presentation of symptoms for a particular patient. Perform an impairment interview in which specific examples of the symptoms are elicited.

Sometimes the symptom will change in one setting but not another. For example, fidgeting may be reduced while playing a game, but not while doing arithmetic homework.

Domains of impairment — Symptoms or behaviors are treated only if they create impairment in the patient's life. The baseline interview elicits specific examples of how the target symptoms affect various domains of functioning. These specific examples provide the concrete situations against which subsequent therapeutic change will be judged. The follow-up interview forms the basis of judgment about the impact of the treatment.

The table at the end of appendix A provides some specific measures of target behaviors known to be treatment-sensitive. These measures have reasonably good empirical support for their use in evaluating dose or time-response effects of medication treatment.

Measuring changes at different medication dosages — To measure changes at different dosages, clinicians should first assess each symptom's impact on school, home, peers, and self, then compare current and initial states of functioning. Be cautious not to mistakenly compare the current state only with a previous patient observation. When clinicians compare the current state with the initial state, they will better document small, incremental changes that occur over time as a result of the medication dosage.

Standardized measures are often used when assessing changes due to therapy. These measures need to be sensitive to treatment effects as well as brief and easy to administer.

What Differentiates ADHD from Other Disorders?

Many normal people experience a decreased tolerance for sitting still, listening, or paying attention to detail. The important difference between these people and those with ADHD is the level of impairment in daily functioning and longevity of the symptoms. For instance, a "squirmy" child who constantly moves in a seat may be able to concentrate and get good grades, or an adult under stress at home may temporarily be forgetful and disorganized at work.

Diagnosing ADHD may be complicated by other conditions with behaviors similar to those typical of ADHD. These other conditions may require interventions different from those for ADHD. Figure 2.6., below, lists both psychiatric and medical conditions for which differentiation must be addressed. **Appendix B covers differential diagnosis in detail.**

Figure 2.6 ADHD Differential Diagnostic Checklist

Psychiatric Disorders	Genetic Disorders	Medical Disorders
✓ Anxiety disorders	✓ Turner syndrome (in females)	✓ Head injury
✓ Bipolar disorder	✓ XYY syndrome (in males)	✓ Dementia
✓ Borderline personality disorder	✓ Fragile X syndrome	✓ Delirium
✓ Oppositional defiant disorder	✓ Neurofibromatosis	✓ Tumors – frontal, parietal, and temporal
✓ Antisocial personality disorder	✓ Treated phenylketonuria (PKU)	✓ Tourette's disorder
✓ Dysthymia and depression (with agitation)	✓ Pervasive developmental disorders (PDD)	✓ Stroke
✓ Post-traumatic stress disorder	✓ Autistic disorder	✓ Hyperthyroidism/hypothyroidism
✓ Histrionic personality disorder	✓ Fetal alcohol syndrome	✓ Renal and hepatic insufficiency
✓ Substance abuse disorders		✓ Anoxic encephalopathy
✓ Intermittent explosive disorder		✓ Vitamin deficiency states
✓ Conduct disorder		✓ Chronic obstructive pulmonary disease
✓ Learning disorders		✓ Multiple sclerosis
		✓ Seizures/epilepsy
		✓ Sensory deficits (e.g., hearing loss)
		✓ Medication side effects
		✓ Neurological disorders of vigilance

* Adapted from Waid & Anton (1998)[126]

Key Concepts for Chapter Two

1. Assessment strategies for ADHD should consider the need to classify someone as eligible for special services (e.g., at school or work) and to determine course of treatment, treatment monitoring, and prognosis.

2. ADHD symptoms **may be expressed differently** at different developmental levels (e.g., a child's inability to sit still could become a tendency to impulsive shopping in adulthood).

3. Establish the presence of symptoms **according to developmental norms** by using well-validated rating scales.

4. Children are typically seen for symptoms of ADHD in middle childhood, when school structure and peer relations place new demands on the child.

5. ADHD symptoms that present only at school may be more representative of a learning disability or challenges with the school environment.

6. **Adolescents** with ADHD tend to be more restless and have more problems with schoolwork than when younger, while adults with ADHD tend to suffer more executive dysfunction (e.g., problems with organization, future planning, and project completion).

7. Obtaining a reliable diagnosis requires applying **all five DSM-IV(TR) criteria**: number of symptoms, age of onset, pervasiveness, impairment, and differential diagnosis.

8. Establish **how the symptoms impair functioning in a particular context** (e.g., home, work, school, with peers, and in mood or self-esteem).

9. A thorough ADHD assessment involves family, psychiatric, developmental, and medical histories as well as patient, parent, and teacher interviews and direct patient observation to understand how the current complaints fit into the patient's "life story."

10. A number of psychiatric, genetic, and medical disorders can present symptoms similar to ADHD. **Differential diagnosis** is critical, especially for depression, dysthymia, bipolar disorder, panic disorder, obsessive-compulsive disorder, or post-traumatic stress disorder.

Chapter Three:
Treating ADHD with Medication

This chapter answers the following:

▶ **What are Stimulant Medications, and How are They Used to Treat ADHD?**
— This section explains the pharmacology of stimulant medications, dose response and time-action, and target behaviors most affected by medications.

▶ **How Safe are Stimulant Medications for Treating ADHD?** — This section addresses side effects, compliance, and contraindications.

▶ **What Options Exist for Other Types of Medication Treatment?** — This section covers non-stimulant and other medication therapies.

▶ **How Effective are Medication Treatments for ADHD?** — This section presents recent findings on the efficacy of using stimulants for children and adults with ADHD.

T REATMENT with medications is the oldest and most thoroughly studied treatment for ADHD. However, successful ADHD medication therapy is a tricky business, involving far more than handing out a pill to someone. Physicians should avoid the knee-jerk response of treating ADHD only with medication in favor of a more comprehensive view of treatment. Some people skip diagnosis and assessment altogether because they falsely believe that if a child responds to a stimulant medication [like Ritalin® (methylphenidate)], he or she must have ADHD.[127] Research shows that even normal children respond positively to stimulant medication, and other psychiatric disorders may also respond to stimulant medications.[128, 129]

Current ADHD treatment involves the use of medications and *psychosocial therapies.* The response to treatment depends on the pattern and severity of symptoms, the family's attitude toward treatment, and the patient's developmental level. This chapter reviews pharmacological treatment, while the next chapter reviews psychosocial and other psychological treatments. Clinicians can access more in-depth coverage of advanced techniques of medical management through resources from several noted experts.[130, 131]

Empirically based expert guidelines are also available. Such guidelines use panels of experts or innovative survey and statistical methods to recommend the latest assessment and treatment approaches.[132, 133]

psychosocial therapies
— therapies that focus on parenting skills, behavior management, education, and social skills

Management of undesirable side-effects is an important aspect of pharmacotherapy and often determines treatment success.

The important elements for understanding how and when to treat ADHD with medications include:

▶ **Pharmacology of the Medication** — Behaviors and bodily functions affected by the medication and medication action on the body

▶ **General Dosing Guidelines** — Clinician practice recommendations for administering stimulants used to treat ADHD

▶ **Dose Response and Time-Action** — Effect of different dosages on bodily functions and actions on the body and brain over time

▶ **Efficacy** — Effect on different target behaviors

▶ **Safety** — Side effects and *toxicity*

▶ **Compliance** — Likelihood of adhering to the medication regimen

▶ **Contraindications** — Important indications for not using medication treatment

toxicity — the level of medication in the body at which point the medication acts as a poison

This chapter concentrates primarily on reviewing stimulant medications, because they have been used the longest and offer both the most effective and safest treatment option. The remainder of the chapter reviews:

▶ Non-stimulant medication treatment

▶ Treating ADHD adults with medications other than stimulants

▶ Effectiveness of medication treatments for ADHD

From the Patient's Perspective

Things seem to be going better. My grades are better at school, and it's a little easier to pay attention. Mom thinks it's because of the pills, but the doctor keeps changing the time of day I take them, so I don't know. They seem to keep checking my weight, and now I get to have a big milkshake every day that's supposed to be good for me and help me gain weight. The doctor wants me to keep taking the pills even though I won't be seeing her very much anymore.

What are Stimulant Medications, and How are They Used to Treat ADHD?

Stimulants are the most frequently used medications for treating ADHD; those currently used include:

► Methylphenidate (Methylin®/Metadate®/Concerta®/Focalin™/Ritalin®)

► Dextroamphetamine (Dexedrine®/DextroStat®)

► Adderall®

All of the medications listed are variants of either amphetamine or methylphenidate. One new medication formulation (dex-methylphenidate or Focalin™) is unique in that it removes the part of the methylphenidate molecule that has little or no effect on the brain and body, which appears to prolong the time course of the medication action.[134, 135]

Stimulant medications differ in the particular medication-delivery method. For example:

► **Concerta®** employs a hard, virtually unbreakable capsule with an ingenious osmotic membrane that allows a precise delivery of the medication over a 12-hour period. Its more immediate effect is achieved with a small amount of an overcoating of immediate-release medication.

► **Metadate CD®** (controlled delivery), **Ritalin LA®** (long-acting), and **Adderall XR®** use tiny beads containing both immediate-release and long-acting components, so the capsule can be broken open and sprinkled on food if necessary.

These different medication-delivery methods affect the *pharmacokinetics* (PK) of the distribution and absorption of the medications in the body, which in turn affects the way the medication acts on the body *pharmacodynamics* (PD). Some patients may do better on one pattern of medication-delivery than another, so these new delivery methods give clinicians more options in finding the right medication for a particular patient.

Pharmacology of Stimulant Medications

The term "stimulant" is an historical label that does not accurately describe the full action of stimulant medications in the brain. Psychostimulants are rapidly absorbed into the brain, with peak blood levels and effects on behavior occurring in one to three hours. While stimulants increase activity in nerve cells in many different parts of the brain, they also cause increased *inhibition*, particularly in the *neocortex* or frontal parts of the brain.

The stimulating or activating effects of these medications produce an alert, focused attention. The inhibitory effects shut out

Pemoline (Cylert®/Pemolert™) is now seldom recommended because of occasional, severe toxicity involving liver function.

*Although the medications are not new, the variety of newer medication **formulations** gives the clinician more flexibility for developing dose-response and time-action curves for each patient (see pages 39–41).*

pharmacokinetics — the mathematics of the time course of absorption, distribution, metabolism, and excretion (ADME) of medications in the body, which aids the clinician's ability to individualize medication therapy

pharmacodynamics — the study of medication action in the body over a period of time, including the processes of absorption, distribution, localization in the tissues, bio-transformation, and excretion

inhibition — a response caused by specific neurotransmitters binding to receptors on a neuron that decreases the probability that neurotransmitters will be released by the neuron

neocortex — the most recently developed and neurologically complex part of the brain

Early studies focused on "hyperactivity" as the main therapeutic target, neglecting the many cognitive and emotional effects caused by widespread brain activation.

dopamine and norepinepherine — chemicals in the brain that help regulate motor-control systems and central nervous system functioning

Over 50 years of research on stimulant treatment of ADHD has found these medications to positively affect a variety of factors, such as:[138]

► *Attention*
► *Impulsivity*
► *Aggression*
► *Defiance*
► *On-task concentration*
► *Disruptive verbal behavior*
► *Social functioning*
► *Memory*

unwanted stimuli or responses. This allows the patient to pay selective attention to appropriate or desired stimuli from among many possible options. Thus, activation is like powering a vehicle, while inhibition is like using the brakes or steering mechanism. The combination of these two effects produces a wealth of changes well beyond a simple lowering of activity level.

The exact biochemical and anatomic mechanisms of stimulants are not entirely understood. They are thought to work primarily by increasing availability of two neurotransmitters or chemicals that allow information to pass from one brain cell to another. These neurotransmitters, *dopamine and norepinephrine*, have an influence on attention, response to rewarding cues, alertness, activity level, and exploratory behavior.

Experts believe dopamine is important for paying attention to interesting environmental cues or those relevant to survival. For example, dopamine may affect the functions that facilitate an infant's ability to recognize its mother's face or voice. Such cues generally cause an approach response. Presumably, a deficit in dopamine functioning will lead to a lack of appropriate activation ("inattention") and a random response to irrelevant stimuli ("hyperactivity").

Norepinephrine affects the response to reward cues, including cues that signal threat, punishment, or non-reward.[136] Since these stimuli usually cause behavioral inhibition, such as stopping and inspecting the environment before acting or approaching, a deficit in norepinephrine functioning will presumably lead to impulsive, daredevil, or heedless responding and a failure to learn how to control impulses. On the other hand, over-responsiveness of this system may lead to excessive behavioral inhibition and anxiety.[137]

Some research supports the role of dopamine and norepinephrine as causal factors in hyperactivity. For example, animal studies indicate that if the dopamine-producing nerves of rats are damaged during early development, the animals become hyperactive and fail to learn. Administering a stimulant medication corrects the deficits.[139] Some of the chemicals produced by these neurotransmitters have been found in body fluids of ADHD patients, especially after treatment with stimulants. However, a variety of other studies fail to confirm the role of neurotransmitters in ADHD.[18]

General Dosing Guidelines

Figure 3.1 on the next page provides an overview of key medications used to treat ADHD as well as common dosage recommendations based on clinical practice. Figure 3.2, on page 42, provides answers to clinicians' most frequently asked questions about medication and dose selection.

Figure 3.1   Stimulants Used in ADHD Treatment

Generic Class (Time Action) (Brand Name)	Daily Dose (mg/kg)	Daily Dosage Schedule*	Typical Dosing Schedule
Amphetamine (Immediate Release) (Dexedrine tablets)	0.3–1.5	2–3 times	5–30 mg 2–3 times/day
Amphetamine (Intermediate Release) (Adderall,® Dexedrine Spansules)		1–2 times	5–30 mg twice daily
Amphetamine (Extended Release) (Adderall XR®)		Once	10–30 mg once daily
Methylphenidate (Immediate Release) (Ritalin®)	0.5–2.0	2–4 times	5–40 mg 2–4 times/day
Methylphenidate (Immediate Release) (Focalin™)	0.25–1.0	2–4 times	2.5–20 mg 2–4 times/day
Methylphenidate (Intermediate Release) (Ritalin SR,® Metadate SR®)	0.5–2.0	1–2 times	10–60 mg 1–2 times/day
Methylphenidate (Extended Release) (Concerta,® Ritalin LA,® Metadate CD®)	0.5–2.0	Once	18–108 mg once daily

* The dosage ranges are **not** those recommended on package inserts by the FDA, but those commonly found in clinical practice.
Note: Table adapted from Wilens, Biederman, et. al. (2002)[140]

Dose Response and Time-Action

Measuring effectiveness of stimulant treatment involves aware-
ness of the types of **dose response curves** and **time-action,** or
how the medication affects targeted behaviors at different times.
Stimulant medications are typically administered one to three times
daily, depending on each specific formulation and packaging.

Dosage Response Curves

Stimulants produce three different types of dose-response
curves that can vary with individuals and the target behaviors
being measured:[141, 142]

> ▶ **Linear Response** — This is the most common response;
> an increasing dose causes increasing improvement.

> ▶ **Threshold Response** — In this response, nothing
> happens at lower doses, then a response kicks in at a
> higher dose.

> ▶ **Quadratic Response** — With this dose response,
> behavior first improves with increasing doses, then
> worsens as doses are raised further.

Different individuals will often have different dose-response
curves. Also, some individuals have one type of curve with
one symptom, but a different curve with another symptom
or behavior. For example, an increase in dose might cause a
linear response in activity level, but a **quadratic response** in

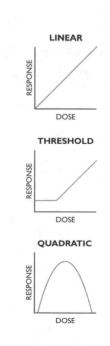

titration — medication
dosage adjustment

memory or attention. Thus, increasing the dose by too much might improve hyperactivity at the cost of poorer memory or attention. Though the general dosages provided in figure 3.1 are useful, each patient's own dose-response curve must be calculated by careful *titration*, while monitoring both learning and behavior.

Common mistakes include under-dosing for the threshold response and linear response types, and overdosing for the quadratic response type. Adequate titration requires knowing which target behaviors change at what dose at a particular point in the time-action curve. This knowledge can only be gained by carefully observing different target behaviors as they respond to a particular dose. Thus, when the clinician gives the lowest dose, (e.g., 5 mg of Ritalin® in the morning), the patient's response to a simple arithmetic test and activity level during the period of peak action (one to two hours) provides the first point on the dose-response curve. By gradually raising the dose to a medium (10 mg) and high level (15 mg) a dose-response curve could be constructed. This might need to be done for several measures or for each target domain. Findings might reveal that at a particular time of day, a certain dose is just fine for activity level but too high for optimal arithmetic performance. (Chapter two offers practical solutions to measuring target behaviors.)

Assessing medication response in adults differs from assessment in children because of the reliance on self-reports. Adults with ADHD are often unaware of their social impact on others and may underestimate treatment effects on family and social relationships. Therefore, clinicians should include reports of significant others, whenever possible, during a medication evaluation.

Since adults often have coexisting depression and low self-esteem, the new non-stimulant atamoxetine (Straterra®), antidepressants, such as bupropion (Wellbutrin®), or the TCAs may be appropriate, since they will also affect these coexisting conditions. However, controlled research has not yet verified this presumption.

For many adults, restlessness or hyperactivity may be less important than the ability to start a task, concentrate on its execution, and finish it in a timely manner without procrastination. A new, standardized rating scale for assessment and treatment monitoring of ADHD in adults is now available and includes forms for the patient and significant other.[35]

Time-Action

Knowing how target behaviors respond at one point in time is not usually adequate for administering stimulants, whose effects can have a very rapid onset and dissipation. To achieve the best result, measure dose effects at several points in time. Medication effects differ at different times of the day, depending on when the clinician first administers the medication and the timing of subsequent doses. New medications extend the time-action of stimulants. These tend to eliminate the peaks and troughs experienced with shorter-acting stimulants.

Factors Impacting Dose Response and Time-Action

Evaluating dose response and time-action effects of a medication involves consideration of several factors:

- ▶ How the medication affects behavioral and cognitive functioning (i.e., taking action vs. thinking)
- ▶ The way parents, teachers, and patients interpret the medication response
- ▶ School policies that affect administering the medication
- ▶ The patient's daily schedule

How the medication affects behavioral vs. cognitive functioning — Research with stimulants indicates short-lived effects on cognitive functions such as attention. On the other hand, the effects on activity level tend to be more sustained.[143] Some researchers believe that the optimal doses required for cognitive and behavioral functions are different, with hyperactivity requiring a higher dose in order to achieve a positive response. This sometimes leads to the problem of increasing the dose to control one behavior (e.g., hyperactivity) at the expense of overdosing cognitive functions (e.g., learning or attention). Overdosing may lead to cognitive or emotional constriction and the "zombie-like personality" that some parents complain of when children take stimulants. The art of stimulant management consists of carefully adjusting the dose and timing of the medication to achieve optimal behavioral **and** optimal cognitive effects.

The way parents, teachers, and patients interpret medication response — Input from teachers and parents may vary. When responses from the school setting are used to adjust the stimulant dose, problems occurring later in the day (e.g., paying attention to homework) may be under-treated. Conversely, when the assessment only considers the parent's observations at the end of the day, overdosing may occur because a parent may be unaware of the behavioral and cognitive responses to lower doses in the classroom setting.

School policies that affect administering the medication — Most schools have a program for administering prescribed medications. Now that long-acting medications are available, much of the problem of administering medication in school can be avoided. However, it is still very important that the physician obtain in-school reports of side effects and efficacy to administer the medications properly.[144, 145]

The patient's daily schedule — In elementary school, most children have important academic work in the morning. Make sure the medication is close to its peak of action during that time. Sometimes parents give the medication at home around 7:00 a.m. and the peak of medication action wears off before the child's reading or math instruction at 2:00 p.m. Target the most pressing areas of need, and make sure the medication is available during that period.

> Cognitive effects are often ignored in the common administration of stimulants because a decreased activity level is more noticeable than a loss of learning or attention.

> Older adolescents and adult patients need to provide feedback regarding the effects of the medication at different times during their daily schedule.

Figure 3.2   Clinicians' Frequently Asked Questions about Using ADHD Medications

Frequently Asked Questions	Treatment Recommendations
Should I start treatment with an amphetamine or methylphenidate?	Of the two, methylphenidate has been the subject of more research studies, but the efficacy and side effects are virtually indistinguishable, and most patients respond equally well to either. Some patients respond well to one but not the other.[146]
Which dose is best for a new patient?	Start with the lowest dose of the medication, and increase it gradually, with changes upward every three to four days, based on feedback from parents and teachers (or the adult patient). Allergic response to stimulants is rare, but safety dictates that especially when dealing with long-acting medications (such as Concerta,® Adderall XR,® or Ritalin LA®), the patient should be given a low dose first. Routine upward titration is not recommended without patient and/or family feedback regarding a given dose.
How do I tell how much medication is too much?	The medication dose should be increased: (a) until the response measure shows no further room for improvement; and (b) side effects are limited and tolerable. When side effects persist over one to two weeks and are severe, the dosage should be dropped down until side effects remit to a tolerable level. If efficacy worsens, then consider another stimulant.
What if the patient only has partial response?	Many patients will respond in one area and fail to respond in another. In such cases, one should consider switching to another stimulant. Only if results are unsatisfactory should one switch to a non-stimulant or add another medication. Combining a stimulant with another stimulant is an emerging pediatric practice option but one for which there is limited empirical evidence.[147]
How do I measure the best dose for a patient?	As described in chapter two, during assessment one should have noted various **specific impairments** resulting from symptoms (e.g., poor school productivity, lack of prosocial behaviors with peers, or poor classroom deportment). Brief teacher and parent rating scales may capture these problems; but if not, then you should record their frequency or severity informally at different doses of the medication. (Chapter two includes a scale for measuring impairment severity.)
Can I supplement long-acting medications?	One can try small doses of a fast-acting medication at the end of the school day to supplement the long-acting medication. This also applies to supplementation of the morning dose when response is not working fast enough.
Can I safely combine different medication classes?	In treatment-refractory and complex cases, it is not uncommon to combine medication classes. For example, a clinician might prescribe both a stimulant for ADHD and an antidepressant for comorbid depression or add clonidine to the stimulant treatment to ameliorate stimulant-induced insomnia.[148]
Can stimulants cause later medication abuse?	Current evidence suggests that stimulants are actually protective against later illicit medication use and substance abuse disorder (SUD).[149]

Linking Stimulant Medications with ADHD Target Behaviors

Controlled research shows that stimulants positively affect many ADHD characteristics, including:[138]

- ► Core symptoms of ADHD, (e.g., hyperactivity, impulsivity, and inattention)

- ► Symptoms characteristic of conduct disorder, (e.g., aggression, lying, stealing, and conflict with the law)[150, 151]

- ► Symptoms typical of oppositional defiant disorder, (e.g., defiance, argumentativeness, noncompliance, and irritability)[152, 153]

- ► Disturbances of classroom behavior and academic functioning, (e.g., off-task behavior, disruptive verbal behavior, and inability to respond to directions)[154, 155]

- ► Problems with mother-child relationships, (e.g., a mother's controlling reactions to her child's noncompliance and off-task behavior and a mother's ratings of home behavior problems)[156, 157]

- ► Social functioning, (e.g., inappropriate peer interactions, antisocial acts, and aggressive behaviors)[158, 159]

- ► Mood improvement, (e.g., anger/hostility and tension/anxiety)[160]

- ► Specific cognitive functions, (e.g., problems with attention, learning, and working memory)[141, 161]

These characteristics are not unique to ADHD, so a positive response to medications in these areas does not necessarily indicate an ADHD diagnosis.

As noted in chapter two, many possible target behaviors exist. To provide complete dose- and time-action information on a particular patient, clinicians must obtain several measures during the course of a day or several measures taken at different dose levels. Measures of activity level, attention, time-on-task, or academic performance need to be rather brief, easily re-administered, sensitive to medication effects, and lacking in practice effects (i.e., improving merely through repetition of the test). New ADHD "index" and short rating forms provide useful tools for brief and frequently administered assessments of medication response.[162, 163]

Stimulants have a reputation for treating "hyperactivity" since their effect on motor behavior is often so dramatic and impressive. However, even in the earliest studies on children in 1937, Charles Bradley noted wide variations in benzedrine's (a cousin of dextroamphetamine) effects on academic productivity, mood, and general demeanor.

ADHD target symptoms will respond to medication treatment in one child but not another. As a result, effective clinical management dictates performing careful individual assessment before administering medication therapy. Chapter two offers information regarding proper diagnosis.

See appendix A for a review of measures that link medications with target behaviors.

How Safe are Stimulant Medications for Treating ADHD?

Stimulants have been used for over 40 years to treat children with ADHD and related symptoms, with methylphenidate being the most widely used stimulant.[146] Despite an unparalleled safety and efficacy record of methylphenidate and amphetamines and approximate equality in various head-to-head comparisons, a few concerns require special mention, including:[164, 165]

> ▶ **Side effects** — Side effects, such as appetite suppression and insomnia, require regular monitoring. Overall, the side effects of methylphenidate and amphetamine are approximately the same in number, though some evidence indicates that insomnia and appetite suppression are more severe for amphetamine.[165]

> ▶ **Compliance** — Many patients fail to take medications as prescribed, which affects successful treatment. Patient intelligence, symptom severity, and family/teacher involvement will affect compliance.[166, 167]

> ▶ **Contraindications** — Some *comorbid* disorders affecting the patient (or the patient's family) dictate caution when using stimulant medications.

At the recommended dosages, most side effects in most children are easily managed and unlikely to require stopping the medication for either class of medications.

comorbid — the simultaneous presence of two or more disorders

Side Effects

Stimulant side effects are usually mild and easily manageable. However, there are many possible side effects because, in addition to their central actions, stimulants produce a variety of effects on the *sympathetic nervous system* and the *parasympathetic nervous system*. The effects on the sympathetic nervous system include:

> ▶ Tachycardia (palpitations or racing heart)

> ▶ Increased blood pressure

> ▶ Other arousal symptoms that often lead to insomnia

The parasympathetic system affects the hypothalamus, a small structure in the brain that regulates appetite, temperature, and other bodily functions. Additional parasympathetic side effects are usually mild and of little consequence, such as stomach upset or headache.

Figure 3.3 on page 46 indicates major side effects and associated management techniques. The following special notes address growth suppression, toxicity, and rebound effects important to clinical management:

sympathetic nervous system — part of the autonomic nervous system that regulates arousal functions, such as dilation of pupils, accelerated heart rate, and adrenaline secretion

parasympathetic nervous system — part of the autonomic nervous system that involves restful state bodily functions such as food digestion

> ▶ **Growth suppression** — Dopamine is important in the regulation of growth hormone and prolactin. At very high doses, stimulants can cause some delay in bone

growth. However, at the recommended doses of stimulants, usually only temporary effects on body weight occur, with no effect on body height.

When dosages are quite high, however, small decreases in linear growth may become permanent. When regular, close monitoring of height suggests that a child is deviating from his or her own established growth curve, the child should have "medication holidays" on weekends or vacations. Children treated with stimulants should be monitored in at least six-month intervals for growth.

In a recent follow-up of the large, multi-site study of ADHD (MTA), covering two years of stimulant medication treatment, researchers found that continuously medicated children (originally seven to nine years of age) grew about .75 of an inch less in height than the normal comparison group and weighed about 8.5 pounds less. When compared to the **national** average, the continuously medicated group grew slightly slower than the national average (about .75 inch less than expected).[168]

These long-term results suggest that clinicians must frequently monitor growth rates and adjust dosage as necessary to minimize slowing of growth. (Since these results are for children medicated prior to their adolescent growth spurt, further data will be required to determine if the slowing persists during the growth-spurt period.)

▶ **Severe toxic effects** — With stimulants, severe toxic effects are rare. A possible exception is the risk of liver complications with pemoline (Cylert®), requiring careful monitoring of liver enzymes at the start of treatment and throughout its course. The possibility that such monitoring may not prevent severe liver complications has led to recent "black box" warnings by the FDA.

▶ **Rebound** — Rebound effect occurs when behavior worsens as the stimulant wears off, sometimes returning to a level greater than usual. Now that long-acting medications are available, there is less concern about a rebound effect.[169, 170] When it does occur, this problem usually happens in the afternoon or near the end of the day as a midday dose wears off. To address the problems, many clinicians add a third dose of a stimulant, usually half that taken at the midday dose. This approach avoids rebound effects and often improves evening social activities or homework concentration.

Research indicates that many children show a temporary suppression of weight gain due to reduced appetite when taking stimulants. However, children usually experience a growth spurt after a short while on the medication, with few children treated actually remaining smaller in stature than expected.

A multimodal treatment study of ADHD, sponsored by the National Institutes of Health, validated treatment success when trained professionals follow specific ADHD treatment protocol manuals. For more information on this study, see appendix C.

Caution: Although the manufacturer no longer markets Cylert,® there are many pemoline generics still available.

Figure 3.3   Managing Side Effects

Side Effect	Recommended Clinical Management
General	• For mild side effects, allow 7 to 10 days for tolerance to develop. • Determine if a lower dose will remove side effects. • Evaluate time-action, and determine if timing of administration can be adjusted to minimize side effects. • Determine whether side effects are related to other disorders or current environmental stressors, and adjust accordingly. • If these strategies fail, consider an alternative stimulant.
Anorexia/ Dyspepsia	• Administer medication before, at, or after a meal. • For pemoline, consider medication-induced hepatitis.
Weight Loss	• Give medication after breakfast or lunch. • Try calorie enhancement strategies, such as high-protein instant breakfasts laced with ice cream. • Get eating started with any highly preferred food before giving regular foods. • Try brief "medication holidays."
Slowed Weight or Height Gain	• Apply weight-loss remedies. • Give longer (weekend or vacation) medication holidays. • Change to another stimulant, or consider a non-stimulant.
Dizziness	• Monitor blood pressure and pulse. • Encourage adequate hydration. • If associated only with peak medication effect, try sustained release preparation.
Insomnia/ Nightmares	• Administer medication earlier in the day. • Omit or reduce last dose. • If taking sustained release, change to tablet. • Consider adding a sedating antihistamine such as benadryl or clonidine.
Dysphoric Mood, Emotional Constriction	• Reduce dose, or switch to long-acting preparation. • Switch stimulants. • Consider comorbid OCD, requiring alternative or adjunctive treatment.
Rebound	• Switch to sustained-release preparation. • Combine sustained-release and short-acting preparations.
Tics	• Conduct medication trial at different doses, including no medication, to be sure tics are medication related. • For mild tics that abate after 7 to 10 days, reconsider risk vs. benefit, and negotiate a new informed consent with the patient/guardian. • Switch stimulants. • Consider nonstimulant treatment, such as clonidine or an antidepressant. • For severe tics in presence of severe ADHD, consider combining stimulant with a high-potency neuroleptic agent.
Psychosis	• Discontinue stimulant treatment. • Assess for presence of a comorbid thought disorder. • Consider alternative treatments.

Compliance

In some studies, as many as 60 percent of children failed to take their prescribed dose of medication.[171] Poor adherents to medication tend to be less intelligent, have more severe symptoms, and achieve lower academic scores than those who adhere to medication schedules.[172] Additionally, parents with undiagnosed ADHD or depression sometimes fail to consistently administer medication.[173] Parent education appears to be the main approach to increasing compliance.

Chaotic households or families with a lack of basic resources are often poor risks for successful medication therapy. As more primary needs take priority, it's unlikely that medication schedules will be followed. Also, observation of side effects and efficacy may be unreliable.

Contraindications

Although stimulants are generally quite safe for children with ADHD, a few conditions in the patient or the patient's immediate family indicate stimulants should be given only with caution, if at all. These include:

- ▶ **Thought disorder or psychosis** — Stimulants can exacerbate a thought disorder, leading to a stimulant-induced hallucinosis. Therefore, stimulants must be used with caution in children evidencing psychotic behavior or who have family histories of schizophrenia or manic-depressive psychosis.

- ▶ **Tourette's Syndrome** — Be cautious when there is a family history of Tourette's syndrome or evidence of vocal and motor tics in the child. Currently, controversy exists as to the likelihood of exacerbating a neurological condition by administering stimulants to patients with Tourette's. However, recent double-blind trials suggest that methylphenidate may actually improve Tourette's symptoms in many patients.[176]

Some have suggested that adults with ADHD and psychosis can be safely treated with stimulants.[174, 175] However, current diagnostic criteria do not allow psychosis as a comorbid disorder for ADHD, and count it as an exclusionary criterion for diagnosis of ADHD.

- ▶ **Substance abuse** — Although early effective treatment with stimulants probably reduces the risk of later substance abuse, adolescents and families who are known substance abusers must be treated with caution.[177] In such circumstances, it may be wise to use one of the medications less likely to be misused, such as Straterra,® or an antidepressant medication.

- ▶ **Liver or cardiac dysfunction** — Children with past histories of liver problems should not take pemoline (previously marketed as Cylert®), and those using it should have regular monitoring of liver function. Because of their effects on the heart, patients with preexisting cardiac problems should be excluded from certain medications.

- ▶ **Coexisting psychiatric conditions** — ADHD is often accompanied by other disorders that require special

***Caution:** Although the manufacturer no longer markets Cylert,® there are many pemoline generics still available.*

treatment consideration. Some of these common coexisting disorders are:

- **Oppositional and aggressive conduct disorder.** Studies indicate that stimulants have a beneficial effect on many of these behaviors.[138]

- **Anxiety and depression.** Some evidence indicates that anxiety lessens the effectiveness of stimulant treatment.[178] But since anxiety and depression have little effect on the ADHD symptom response to tricyclic antidepressants, these are a good choice when anxiety and depression are present.

- **Obsessive-compulsive disorder.** Specialized treatment is required for this disorder, which may worsen with stimulant treatment alone or may require other medication along with a stimulant.

- **Learning disorders.** These disorders are very common in ADHD patients. Although stimulants can be helpful, educational intervention is almost always required as well.

What Options Exist for Other Types of Medication Treatment?

Although 60 to 80 percent of children respond well to fast-acting, immediate release stimulants, alternative medication treatment may be necessary for several reasons, including:

- Lack of efficacy at all doses
- Persistent or severe side effects
- A complicating, coexisting disorder that requires non-stimulant treatment

The most common reason for lack of efficacy of a stimulant is failure to provide an adequate dosage or failure to try another stimulant.[179] However, when these reasons do not apply, consider treatment with an antidepressant medication.

Non-Stimulant Medications

Non-stimulant medications used (typically as alternatives) when stimulant treatment is unsuccessful include:

- Atomoxetine (Straterra®)
- Some tricyclic antidepressants
- Bupropion (Wellbutrin®)
- Selective serotonin reuptake inhibitors (*SSRIs*)
- Clonadine (Catapres®)

Combined use of antidepressants and stimulants requires close monitoring to prevent toxicity since methylphenidate interferes with metabolism of the tricyclics.[180]

SSRIs — medications that slow down the ability of nerve cells to absorb serotonin, a neurotransmitter

▶ Guanfacine (Tenex®)

▶ Some anticonvulsants

▶ Venlafaxine (Effexor®)

The newly-approved medication, **atomoxetine (Straterra®),** is a non-stimulant that appears to be a very specific re-uptake blocker of norepinephrine, in contrast to the stimulants that appear to largely act through dopamine neurotransmitter reuptake blocking.

See page 38 for information on the role of norepinephrine, dopamine, and reuptake blocking in ADHD.

Recent clinical trials show that atomoxetine is safe, and is superior to placebo for children, adolescents, and adults. Because of its relatively recent use, long-term exposure data will be important for the acceptance of this agent as a confirmed member of the pharmacopoeia for ADHD.

As a non-stimulant, this medication may be more palatable to patients or families for whom the term "stimulants" carries bad connotations (despite their long use and good track record of efficacy and safety).

Tricyclic antidepressant medications (TCAs), such as imipramine, desipramine, and nortriptyline, are proven effective (especially in adults) and reasonably safe for those with ADHD.[181] These medications have a much slower onset of action than stimulants do and require adequate blood levels before the effect becomes noticeable. Therefore, clinicians must exercise more patience in detecting beneficial effects before altering the therapy. Evidence suggests that though effective, these medications are less effective than stimulants, and desipramine should be avoided because of its greater toxicity.[182]

TCAs require close monitoring because of potentially lethal cardiovascular toxicity.

Bupropion (Wellbutrin®) is an antidepressant with a demonstrated, beneficial effect on ADHD children and adolescents, though controlled trials differ on whether or not it is as effective as the stimulants.[183, 184]

SSRI antidepressants (e.g., Prozac®) are frequently used either alone or in combination with stimulants, but further research is essential on the efficacy, safety, and pharmacokinetics of these medications in children and adolescents.[185]

Clonidine (Catapres®) and guanfacine (Tenex®) are two other medications that clinicians sometimes recommend, especially for children with ADHD who also have tics or who are aggressive, explosive, excitable, or hard to get to sleep. However, the empirical evidence for the efficacy of these medications is from small, poorly controlled trials; further research is needed before knowing which patients should be treated with these medications, and whether they can be recommended without qualification. Concerns have been expressed recently regarding the lethal toxicity of clonidine used in combination with methylphenidate.[187]

Some research suggests that clonidine may be particularly useful in ADHD with comorbid disorders.[186]

Anticonvulsants, such as Depakote,® Tegretol,® Carbatrol,® and Klonopin,® are sometimes used when other medications fail or when there is an extremely aggressive and irritable pattern of behavior. The evidence for their efficacy is very limited, and side effects can be significant.

Venlafaxine (Effexor®) has some evidence from an uncontrolled trial of efficacy in ADHD, with positive effects on behavior but not on cognitive function.[188]

The pharmaceutical industry is actively researching new compounds for ADHD or investigating application of old medications. Current efforts involve exploring medications to be developed from entirely new molecules or from medication classes not usually associated with ADHD.

For example, findings that nicotine may benefit adults with ADHD is prompting research on medications that target nicotinic receptors in the brain. [189–191]

How Effective are Medication Treatments for ADHD?

Research indicates effective results with a variety of other medications used to treat ADHD such as tricyclic antidepressants.[138] However, these results are usually of a lesser magnitude than those targeting stimulant medication treatment.

Thousands of research studies have documented the effectiveness of stimulants for children with ADHD. Reviews of this research consistently attest to the benefits.[192] These studies generally show that the medications are effective in reducing a variety of problem behaviors. Effects on overt behavior have usually been much larger than effects on cognitive problems or academic performance. However, most studies find that cognitive processing also improves (e.g., speed of information handling, accuracy, time-on-task, selective or sustained attention).

In contrast, relatively few, well-controlled stimulant or other trials have been undertaken with adult sufferers of ADHD. The following addresses available results for both children and adult research studies.

Efficacy Research in Children

Most studies of stimulant efficacy in children are of short duration (i.e., three to four months) because of significant problems in carrying out long-term controlled research.[193]

The milestone Multimodal Treatment Approach (MTA) study, sponsored by the National Institute of Mental Health (NIMH) and the U.S. Department of Education, was conducted over 14 months at multiple sites using multiple treatment approaches.[168]

standard treatment in the community — treatment initiated by parents and chosen from a list of physicians, psychologists, and other mental health providers not affiliated with the research study

This study compared treatments of stimulant medication alone, psychosocial therapy alone, stimulant medication and psychosocial therapy combined, and patient-selected community treatment *(standard treatment in the community)*.

Study results related to medication indicate the following:

▶ Stimulant medication treatment, using systematic titration and careful monitoring, was equivalent to combined therapy, and superior to the other two treatment groups in reducing ADHD core symptoms of inattention, hyperactivity/impulsivity, and oppositional-defiant symptoms (e.g., aggression and conduct problems). These effects were apparent in both teacher and parent rating scales as well as in direct classroom observations

▶ Patient's experienced greater reduction in ADHD symptoms when treated by specially trained professionals following specific ADHD treatment protocol manuals.

▶ Patients receiving carefully titrated medication treatment based in medication *algorithms* fared better than those in community treatment plans.

▶ Clinicians' frequent contacts with parents and teachers improved compliance to medication treatment and outcome. Close involvement and feedback to parents and teachers appears essential.

▶ Taking medications on weekends improved outcome.[194]

The MTA study supports previous findings indicating that ADHD medication treatment involves complex algorithms to guide individual titration and that non-expert pharmacotherapy may lead to poor results.[195] Some researchers argue, however, that almost 100 percent of patients respond if dosages are pushed high enough and more than one stimulant is tried.[179]

Poor response to medication treatment can occur because:

▶ Intolerable side effects, such as sustained insomnia, loss of appetite, or stomach complaints, increase the likelihood that patients will not take medications as prescribed. Additionally, this situation makes higher dosages unrealistic in extended treatment situations.

▶ Up to 30 percent of children are non-responders to stimulant or other medication treatments.[34]

▶ Partial responders, who experience improvement in some symptoms or domains of functioning, often experience a lack of improvement in other, sometimes crucial, areas (e.g., academic or social skills).

▶ Medication effects may decrease during the second year of treatment for all age groups (improvements in relationships noticed at the beginning of treatment tend to fade over time).

algorithms — rule-based systems for making decisions

Appendix C describes MTA study design, results after 14 months, and treatment outcomes after 24 months.

Efficacy Research in Adults

In an early review of medication trials, response to treatment varied between 25 and 78 percent. However, with careful diagnostic methodology, confirmed childhood onset of the illness, and robust doses of a stimulant, response was comparable to that in childhood.[138]

In a more recent review of adult trials, there was evidence for the efficacy of amphetamines from five studies (four controlled, one open). However, methylphenidate data from six, controlled trials were conflicting: three studies indicate efficacy, while two studies fail to show such efficacy, possibly due to methodological reasons. The results from the sixth study were equivocal.[196]

Although, there is only limited data currently available, **antidepressants** possibly may offer an effective therapy for adult ADHD. Controlled trials have studied desipramine, atomoxetine (Straterra®), and bupropion (Wellbutrin®), with most evidence supporting the efficacy of desipramine. The initial data from the MTA, 14-month trial indicates that atomoxetine is less effective than desipramine. The efficacy of bupropion is unclear. Initial published open data suggest a response rate of 50–78 percent with venlafaxine.[197]

moderating factors — features at baseline that affect outcome

mediating factors — factors that affect the outcome of the trial that is underway.

Subsequently, there have been several important additional findings during the two- to three-year period of analyses and follow-up data collection. New analyses explore new outcome measures; the **predictors of outcome;** the role of *moderating factors* and *mediating factors*, such as initial severity and subsequent medication history. These findings are currently submitted for publication and not yet available in published form.

The success of medication therapy for ADHD treatment has often preempted the important role of other therapies. The following chapter highlights these other therapies as necessary approaches in a comprehensive treatment approach to ADHD.

Key Concepts for Chapter Three

1. The clinician needs to establish, measure, and regularly reevaluate treatment targets using reliable scales or observations. Successful strategies for achieving those targets require evaluating the pharmacology of the medication, dosing guidelines, dose-response and time-action curves, efficacy, safety, compliance, contraindications, and outcomes.

2. Stimulant medications have been used the longest and appear to be the safest and most effective treatments for ADHD.

3. Since stimulants differ in their medication delivery methods, clinicians need to individualize medication treatment.

4. Clinicians must calculate each patient's dose-response curve through careful titration as well as monitoring of impacts on learning and behavior. Additionally, time-action should be measured at several points during the day.

5. For children, how adults interpret their response to medication, school routines, and policies about giving medications at school all impact does-response and time-action evaluations.

6. Despite the safety and efficacy record of stimulants, concerns over side effects, compliance, and contraindications have led to the development of alternative medication treatments used alone or in combination with stimulant medications.

7. The MTA study found that stimulant medication treatment was most effective when:

   ■ Used with systematic titration (based in medication algorithms) and careful monitoring

   ■ Administered by specially trained clinicians following specific ADHD treatment protocols

   ■ Accompanied by frequent contact between clinicians and parents/teachers to ensure compliance

   ■ Administered on weekends as well as during the week

8. It is important to treat coexisting conditions along with the core ADHD disorder.

Chapter Four:
Psychological Treatments for ADHD

This chapter answers the following:

▶ **Why are Medications Alone Not Enough?** — This section covers areas of functional impairment not addressed by medication treatment and presents reasons for using psychosocial treatments.

▶ **What Psychotherapies are Most Often Used to Treat Children with ADHD?** — This section focuses on behavioral and cognitive treatment methods and addresses how other traditional psychotherapeutic approaches have been used to treat ADHD.

▶ **How Effective is a Multimodal Therapy Approach?** — This section summarizes key results from research on patients treated with both psychotherapy and medication.

▶ **What Psychological Treatments are Used for Treating Adults with ADHD?** — This section explores psychoeducation, coaching, and environmental restructuring as well as behavioral management, cognitive, and relaxation techniques.

Why are Medications Alone Not Enough?

STIMULANTS and other medications powerfully treat ADHD. Although much evidence supports the value of medication, there are several important reasons why psychological treatments may be needed for ADHD, either by themselves or in combination with medication.[198, 199] These treatments are helpful because some children:

▶ Fail to respond to medication therapy even if it is well managed

▶ Have a partial response but still have important symptoms not managed by the medication (often because of coexisting conditions or environmental complications)

▶ Experience severe side effects or toxicity, which limit the usefulness of medication therapy

▶ Undergo developmental changes that may require new treatment strategies

Psychological treatments are also helpful because some parents:

▶ Have fundamental objections to medicating children, either because of attitudinal, religious, or other reasons

▶ Can improve important treatment outcomes by changing parenting practices and cognitions

▶ May themselves be impaired from ADHD or other psychiatric conditions, which must be alleviated for the child's treatment to be effective

Medications are excellent treatments for removing symptoms, but they may be insufficient for teaching new skills. Building positive habits or skills may be more effective than trying to suppress unwanted behaviors.

While some treatments may remove symptoms, they may have no effect on learning to acquire new skills. Functional areas requiring new skills for both the patients and their families are social adjustment, negative behaviors and thoughts, academic skills deficits, and parental/family stress reduction.

Social Adjustment

Social adjustment is perhaps the most important area of function in determining successful, long-term outcomes for ADHD children. Research on boys with social disabilities indicates that: [200]

- ▶ They experience much higher rates of mood, anxiety, disruptive, and substance abuse disorders.

- ▶ Baseline social disability in boys with ADHD is a significant predictor of later conduct disorder and most substance abuse disorders.

- ▶ Even after controlling baseline mood and conduct disorders, aggressive behavior, and attention problems, findings are the same.

ADHD is associated with a variety of social problems, including interpersonal acts that are inept, irritating, immoderate, aggressive, or intense.[201]

Children with ADHD are often isolated and rejected early in life. Because they have fewer positive social interactions than other children, they often fail to initiate and sustain social relationships. Though medication may make a child less impulsive in social situations, it may still be difficult for the child to make new friends or remain part of a peer group.

There is little doubt that, with effective medication treatment, children with ADHD may become more manageable at home and show reduced aggressive and non-compliant behavior. Such changes certainly lessen parental criticism or nagging, but teaching positive parenting and reward techniques is needed to build the child's positive behaviors.[202]

Negative Behaviors and Thoughts

Children develop negative behaviors and thoughts in response to failures caused by scattered attention, hyperactivity, or impulsive behavior. *Negative self esteem* is one of the most important of these reactions.[203] Learned through years of failure and rejection, most children's self esteem does not improve following successful medication treatment.[204]

negative self esteem — overall negative beliefs and feelings people have about themselves

Although cognitive-behavioral therapy focuses on negative cognitions about the self, effectiveness trials have been disappointing.[205, 206] Thus improved self-esteem appears to solely arise from effective behavior, not from coaching or praise. However positive praise for effective behavior can lead to improved self-esteem if it encourages the child to engage in more of the effective behavior that earned the praise.

Academic Skills Deficits

Research shows that about 20 percent of children with ADHD also have a learning disability or a deficit in academic skills.[207] Up to 80 percent of children with ADHD (seen at community clinics) suffer academic skills deficits.[208] Though medications enhance some learning and achievement scores, often the effect is not enough. Some research indicates that behavioral treatments are better at addressing academic skills deficits than medication treatment.[209]

Meta-analysis of medication therapy over four decades shows that medication effects on academic measures are significantly smaller than effects on behavior and deportment.[146] Recent data from a large, multi-site, controlled trial of medication versus combined medication plus comprehensive behavioral treatments (the MTA study), shows that children's academic skills improved most when they received behavioral treatment along with medication.[168, 210]

Parental/Family Stress Reduction

Family stress is a complex condition contributed to by both parents and children. The Parenting Stress Index strongly predicts both the child's *oppositional-defiant behavior* and *maternal psychopathology*.[211, 212] Thus, treatment of both the child and parent may actually enhance medication effectiveness over the long term. ADHD creates considerable stress in parents, and highly stressed parents tend to be inattentive to providing consistent and positive consequences for their children's behavior.[213] Therefore, reducing parental stress through parent training might give parents more effective control over their child's behavior. Medication therapy also tends to decrease symptoms that annoy parents. Thus, teaching parents positive behavior control to use along with medication therapy is the approach most likely to succeed.

oppositional-defiant behavior — angry, argumentative, resentful, spiteful, and/or vindictive behaviors

maternal psychopathology — mental and/or behavioral disorders of the mother

From the Patient's Perspective

The doctor helped me not get mad so fast; now, I don't fight with my friends so much. I've been on this reward program at home, which isn't too bad. I get points for finishing my homework and doing stuff like taking out the trash. I can trade in my points for money and time to play video games at the mall. Things are way better, both at school and at home!

What Psychotherapies are Most Often Used to Treat Children with ADHD?

Following an introduction to behavioral and cognitive approaches, this section focuses on the ADHD psychotherapies most often used with children, including:

- ► Direct contingency management (pages 61–62)
- ► Parent training (pages 62–65)
- ► Classroom behavior management (pages 65–67)
- ► Academic skills therapy (page 67)
- ► Social skills therapy (pages 67–68)
- ► Other traditional psychotherapies, such as family therapy and psychodynamic/developmental therapy (page 69)

A later section (pages 71 though 73) addresses psychological treatment strategies for adults with ADHD.

The Behavioral Approach to Treating ADHD

There are many different forms of behavioral therapy. However, only parent training and classroom intervention have proven effective for ADHD.[215] Using rigorous, evidence-based criteria, these approaches clearly offer significant benefits, especially when combined. The combination of these approaches is often referred to as clinical behavior management. These two forms of therapy are actually very similar in their concepts, differing mainly in their adaptation to the specific environment in which they are used.

Common to most behavioral approaches is a functional assessment of the factors that precede the behavior, the specific behaviors that occur in the situation, and the consequences that follow the behavior. This approach is sometimes referred to as the "A-B-C sequence," or Antecedents, Behaviors, and Consequences. For a behavior to occur, certain **antecedents** (conditions, stimuli, or circumstances) must precede or elicit the **behavior**. Whether the behavior increases, stays the same, or decreases depends on the **consequences** that follow the behavior. Behavior theory does not typically concern itself with the inner thoughts, feelings, or motivations, but with the behavior itself. Whether a child "likes" or "doesn't like" a particular consequence is not as important as the likelihood that the behavior will recur.

Positive Reinforcement

This type of reinforcement occurs when consequences that follow behaviors act to increase behaviors. For example, if a child sitting quietly in a chair receives praise from a parent, causing the child to sit quietly more often, then sitting quietly was positively reinforced by the praise. Similarly, if a child is screaming, and attention (by commenting or yelling) increases the screams, then positive reinforcement has also occurred. "Paying attention" to unwanted behavior is often an inadvertent reinforcement in the classroom and at home.

Noncompliance is often inadvertently reinforced because the parent may try to reason with the child, comfort them, or provide attention in other ways. Attention, for the child, is often very rewarding, so the child may perform unwanted behaviors to get attention. This is why one of the first skills taught in parent training is how and when to give a child positive attention.

Negative Reinforcement

Like positive reinforcement, negative reinforcement also increases behavior. But in this case, the consequence is something that is taken away, and its absence increases the behavior. For example, a parent tells a child to stop hitting his sibling, the child fails to comply, whereupon the parent stops giving the command, resulting in the child increasing his hitting.

Punishment

Punishment means that the unwanted behavior is suppressed by painful consequences. In behavior therapy, a particular form of punishment is *response cost*. The response "costs" the subject something, such as earnings or privileges. For example, phone privileges may be taken away from a teenager if he or she comes home late. If either the frequency or degree of late arrivals decreases, loss of phone privileges functions as an effective punishment. However, some punishments only serve to temporarily stop the behavior and often aggravate the situation by increasing anger and rage. Therefore, punishment techniques must be very carefully and selectively applied. Usually results are best, especially for aggressive behaviors, when a combination of positive reinforcement and response cost is used. For example, combine praising being on time (positive social reinforcement) with losing earnings for being late (response cost).

response cost — a form of punishment in which something important is taken away after an undesired behavior takes place

Most parents and teachers remember to punish when an unwanted behavior occurs, but they forget to "catch the child being good" and reward acceptable behavior.

Time Out

This approach removes a child from a reinforcing environment to another, less-rewarding environment for a designated period of time. Common examples include making a child sit on a kitchen chair or sending a child to his room. Although time out is intended only to change the stimuli in the child's immediate environment, children generally view it as a punishment or a painful, unwanted consequence of behavior. Incorrectly applied, time out can become positive or negative reinforcement. For instance, a parent lecturing a child before or after a time out may be rewarding, while time out from difficult or "boring" schoolwork may increase misbehavior.

A key feature of effective time out is requiring the child to perform appropriately when the time out is over, followed by reinforcement (such as praise) for doing the job well. For example, if a parent tells the child to pick up his or her toys, and the child refuses, time out may be an appropriate consequence. But, unless the parent requires the child to complete the command after release from time out, and rewards the child for his or her effort, the time out may further irritate and motivate the child's noncompliance.

Extinction

Generally, extinction works best when combined with positive reinforcement for replacing an old behavior with a new one.

Like punishment, extinction decreases behavior. It is a process of ignoring a behavior (not providing any reinforcement) until it stops completely. For example, when parents ignore a child's temper tantrum, and the tantrum eventually stops, the likelihood of future tantrums decreases. However, parents and teachers must be aware that before the behavior tapers off and eventually decreases, there is often a "response burst" (or dramatic increase in the undesired behavior) for a short period of time.

The Cognitive Approach to Treating ADHD

Cognitive treatment goals involve increasing the patient's ability to solve problems and monitor his or her own behavior.

Cognitive theories emphasize reinforcement principles to alter thoughts or cognitions related to ADHD behaviors. These theories focus on the way internalized speech serves to regulate behavior.[216] "Irrational" or "distorted" thoughts can result in misbehavior. For example, a child who interrupts a game before her turn may be thinking, "The others are taking too long; it's not fair." Changing the child's thoughts or "self-talk" to something more realistic, such as "I know I get impatient; I need to wait my turn," will help control her behavior. Cognitive interventions in the treatment of ADHD are used most often in conjunction with behavioral strategies. Used alone, there is little evidence of their effectiveness.[206, 215] Even in combination with medication, cognitive approaches appear to offer little additional benefit for social skills, academic functioning, or dosage requirements of the medication.[217]

Treatment Methods Using the Behavioral and Cognitive Approaches

Most behavior programs train parents and teachers to alter consequences in order to increase adaptive, on-task behaviors and minimize intrusive, disruptive behaviors.

The most effective ADHD psychological treatments rely heavily on behavioral methods. However, cognitive interventions and other forms of therapy are often added to the behavioral treatments to address symptoms more complex than single behaviors. **Cognitive-behavioral therapy** (CBT) combines approaches for dealing with a wide array of symptoms.

Treatment methods used with CBT add a more complex set of methods and address a wider spectrum of impairment than those methods that focus on a single target behavior. For example, parent training teaches parents the rules of reinforcement, punishment, and time out. Parents then act as behavior managers of the children across many settings, taking a role in school performance and home-based reward programs.

Social skills training works directly to alter the social interactions and competencies of the child with ADHD. Behavioral and cognitive therapies include:

- ► Direct contingency management
- ► Parent training
- ► Classroom behavior management
- ► Academic skills therapy
- ► Social skills therapy
- ► Multimodal therapy

Direct Contingency Management

Direct contingency management applies behavior therapy to particular target behaviors. In this approach, a target behavior response to an intervention is tracked in a systematic way. Contingency management treatment methods can be applied in public, in the home, or in the classroom.

Figure 4.1   Direct Contingency Management System Components

Requirements	Typical examples/notes
Identifying target behaviors	Increasing homework completion, increasing chore completion, or raising a hand before speaking
Determining the reinforcement frequency necessary for behavioral change	Daily, hourly, or when each chore is given
Pinpointing appropriate reinforcers	Fifteen minutes of one-on-one time with a parent each night or earning a point toward receiving a special toy
Explaining the program to the child and beginning reinforcement	
Being consistent	
Keeping track of the target behavior by recording its frequency or duration	Count the times the child initiated homework on his or her own or the length of time spent doing it
Evaluating effectiveness	Conducting periodic reviews to determine when a goal has been reached, what new goals can be added, or which reinforcers need to be changed **Note:** Reinforcers often "wear out" or lose value in altering the behavior. They may need to be exchanged or increased in value
Giving each reinforcement program a seven-week trial before determining success or failure	Expect behavior to possibly get worse before seeing improvement

Behavioral family therapy may involve all family members of the patient.

Figure 4.1 covers components common to direct contingency management systems.

One important, direct contingency management program uses a daily report card. In this approach, teachers fill out a one-page form each day covering specific classroom behavioral targets. After establishing a "menu" of rewards in collaboration with parents, children can bring the report home each day to redeem any earned reward.[207, 218]

These programs typically focus on adults in the child's environment and consult with the children only to identify appropriate reinforcers.

Poor implementation of
contingency management
may account for some of
the reported failures of
this approach.[107]

Educational Components of
parent training include:
1. Learning about ADHD
2. Focusing on parent/child
   relationships
3. Improving
   communication skills
4. Understanding behavior
   management principles

A recent meta-analysis showed that, according to well-designed studies during the past 25 years, contingency management proved to be highly effective in managing ADHD behaviors in the classroom.[219] Increasingly, practitioners recommend contingency management as the treatment of choice for milder cases of ADHD.[107]

Parent Training

Parent training teaches parents how to manage and influence a child's behavior. It employs all of the behavioral principles from direct contingency management and focuses on educational components such as:

1. **Learning about ADHD** — This part of the training involves discussing ADHD symptoms, possible causes, and treatment. Though trainers emphasize the multi-dimensional causes of ADHD, they focus on viewpoints that stress biological and inborn temperament causes. In this approach, parents learn to manage and cope with a chronic disability rather than feeling guilty about a child's behavior.

2. **Focusing on parent/child relations** — This focus addresses the effects of the child's actions and tempera-ment on the parents as well as the parents' actions and temperaments on the child. For example, when attempts to change a child's disruptive behavior are unsuccess-ful, the parents may feel that "Nothing helps," "He will never change," or "She does it on purpose because she knows how mad I get." These thoughts and feelings can profoundly affect the parent/child relationship. Parents often benefit from discussing these feelings because they find out that they are not alone in their struggles. During this phase of parent training, cognitive techniques are often utilized, such as:

   ■ Analyzing irrational thoughts (e.g., "He should remember to do his chores without me telling him.")

   ■ Looking for evidence that disputes those thoughts (e.g., "He sometimes remembers to do his chores, and he doesn't forget on purpose.")

   ■ Reframing the situation or thinking about it from a different perspective (e.g., "Would I want to clean up garbage rather than play?")

   Additionally, clinicians pay attention to how stressful the child's chronic disability can be for the family, how the family copes with these stresses, and how the situation affects various family relationships.

3. **Improving communication skills** — Parents learn to communicate feelings and requests to children without creating conflict. For example, a parent might say, "I don't like it when you yell to get my attention, and so I will ignore you. What I would like you to do is tap me on my arm." Clear communication skills include direct, specific descriptions of the desired behavior and potential consequences for the child rather than merely criticizing the child's problem behavior. This also helps parents clarify what is important.

Parents learn how to make simple and clear requests of their children, such as "In ten minutes, you will need to go to bed," instead of "You need to go to bed soon."

4. **Understanding behavior management principles** — This education focuses on how a parent's response to behavior either increases or decreases desired behaviors. It is based on the behavioral principles outlined on pages 58–60. Parents receive training in:

Training in behavior management principles focuses on increasing attending skills, reinforcing behavior, using reinforcers, and using time out.

■ **Increasing attending skills.** Parents must learn positive and reinforcing techniques early in treatment. Most have developed harsh or negative parenting styles while attempting to manage frustrating ADHD behavior. Because attending skills are critical in shaping children's behavior, this area of behavior management training involves altering the manner in which parents pay attention to their children. Important attending skills include listening, providing positive attention, and ignoring *benign* behavior. During therapy, parents may be asked to attend to the child while the child does an activity. This provides an opportunity for parents to learn how to attend to their child without interfering or asking questions, and how to comment in a positive rather than negative way.

benign — mild, harmless

To listen effectively, parents need to spend time talking and paying attention to positive aspects without correction, direction, or suggestion. This allows a child to feel noticed and appreciated without any potentially negative interactions. These skills are generally difficult, and parents may need considerable practice before they become more comfortable at "just attending."

Using observation, clinicians find that many parents who believe that they regularly engage in attending skills actually direct or guide their child in some manner during these sessions.

Training in positive attention helps parents look for and focus on positive behaviors they want their child to increase or continue. Desirable behaviors need to be noticed more frequently than the child's disruptive behaviors. For example, parents would be asked to pay attention when their child readily complies with a request to get ready for bed. Parents may be required to interrupt their own activities in order to reinforce compliance. A common mistake of parents unskilled in behavioral principles is to take good behavior for granted while noticing virtually every instance of negative behavior.

Positive attention entails learning to look for (or attend to) desirable behaviors rather than being "on the lookout" for problems. Two positive behaviors should be noticed for every negative behavior.

When parents ignore unacceptable benign behavior, they are practicing the behavioral principle of extinction. For example, when children whine to get what they want, parents can simply ignore the whining. Parents should then respond positively when a child asks for something in a more acceptable manner. Over time, whining will subside if reinforcement only occurs for appropriate behavior.

■ **Reinforcing behavior.** This area focuses on parents consciously rewarding desired behaviors and discouraging unwanted ones. These desired behaviors should be broken down into components of overall goals. For example, if the overall goal is to comply with rules, components might involve completing specific chores and adhering to a prescribed bedtime routine.

■ **Using reinforcers.** Clinicians identify appropriate reinforcers for each target behavior and generally divide these reinforcers into reinforcement or punishment (i.e., those that increase positive behavior vs. those that discourage a target behavior). The choices are limitless. Positive reinforcers or rewards can be as basic as food or as complex as earning points for privileges. Punishment may involve the withdrawal of privileges, a requirement to complete extra chores, or a loss of points related to earning money or some other positive reinforcer. Reinforcement requires consistent application. Each behavioral incident or time interval must be recognized. More complex systems may use charts, points, or stars for measuring target behaviors.

Reinforcers may need to be changed periodically to maintain motivation. In addition, target behaviors need to be reinforced frequently enough so that the child experiences success. Two or three target behaviors can be modified at the same time. Before adding new goal behaviors, the child needs to have consistent success with the previous goal behaviors.

■ **Using time out.** Parents learn that time out must be applied consistently and is more effective with preset lengths of time and locations. One reminder may be given as a cue to the child. Parents learn how to handle tantrums that occur when applying time out. Most importantly, after the time out is over, the child must correctly perform and be rewarded for the behavior that initiated the time out.

An example of time out would be when a child fails to comply with a command after a clear warning

Behaviors targeted for modification must be specific, clear, and measurable.

Reinforcers must be important to the child. Some children may not care whether they can stay up late; thus, the privilege has no power to change behavior.

statement (e.g., "If you don't pick up the toys, you will have a time out.") If the child fails to comply, then time out is enforced. After time out, the command would be issued again. When the child complies, the parent must remember to reward correct performance (e.g., "I really like the way you put your toys away — good job!").

Parent training is an essential part of ADHD management, particularly over long periods and as an addition to medication.[220] Parent training has demonstrated effectiveness in reducing parenting stress and increasing parents' self esteem. Research shows that this increase in parental self esteem has a positive impact on the child's ADHD symptoms.[221]

The most common use of parent training is to combine it with a comprehensive behavior management program.[108]

Classroom Behavior Management

There are a wide array of interventions used in school for children with ADHD.[219] Although similar to home-based training programs, classroom behavior management often targets different behaviors. For example, teachers may want to reinforce behaviors, such as remaining in a seat, bringing appropriate materials to class, or raising a hand before talking. Specific techniques found useful with ADHD include:[222, 223]

In classroom behavior management, elements of parent training, behavior management, and cognitive therapies may be employed in a single program.

▶ **Contingency management** (see pages 61–62) — This treatment most often targets annoying or disruptive behavior or increasing positive social behavior. The teacher's attention, positive and negative, becomes a form of reinforcement.

▶ **Modifying antecedent conditions** — Changing the setting or the activity that precedes disruptive behavior or poor attention can be very effective. Modifying the teaching style to fit with the patient's strength of learning can help. For example, teachers can present material verbally for a highly verbal student or use action-oriented examples for a highly physical student.[16]

Modifying the physical classroom environment is another example of modifying antecedent conditions. Students with ADHD often work better when seated towards the front of the room, where they are less distracted by classmates, or near the teacher, where they can receive more reinforcement for appropriate behavior.

▶ **Token economies** — Token economies use both reinforcement and response cost (see pages 58–59), with students earning or losing special privileges through their behavior. To coordinate this behavior management, teachers may develop a daily report card that they send home with the child, using a point system, checks, or stars to communicate school behavior and goal completion to parents. Based on the report card, parents can positively reinforce the child's success at school through verbal praise or other rewards. Having the child consistently bring the report card to and from school often becomes a primary goal in itself.

Methods combining home and school programs are particularly helpful with token economies, allowing parents to reinforce specific academic or classroom behaviors.

▶ **Time out from reinforcement** — Careful attention to time out is important. For example, removing children from tasks they don't like may actually reinforce inappropriate behavior. Conversely, removing a child from rewarding or pleasing activities for inappropriate behavior can be a very effective intervention.

Teachers often complain that, "I tried time out, and it never worked." Examination of the classroom environment may show that it is not a rewarding environment. In fact, classroom studies show that many teachers give an excess of negative discipline compared to positive (or rewarding) reinforcement.

self-talk — a strategy of talking oneself through a problem or task either silently or aloud

▶ **Cognitive behavioral strategies** — Some specific cognitive strategies useful for ADHD are *self-talk* and repeating instructions. As an example, suppose a child watches a teacher complete a math problem. As the teacher works, he or she uses positive self-talk saying, "Keep trying; remember it takes time to get it right." The teacher may also verbalize step-by-step directions to complete the problem, such as: "Now, I need to carry the number here, then put in the decimal point." The child then attempts a problem with directions and positive feedback from the teacher. Over time, the child begins to make these types of statements with decreased prompts from the teacher. Eventually, the child uses these techniques spontaneously while doing class work.

peer tutoring — having another student work one-on-one with the student with ADHD

▶ **Peer tutoring** — *Peer tutoring* is a promising method to increase students' academic skills.[223] With this approach, a classmate helps the child with ADHD go through a reading, math, or spelling lesson while providing encouragement and direction. Those with ADHD often have difficulty simultaneously taking notes and listening to the material during classroom instruction. In these cases, a classmate can be assigned as a "buddy note-taker."

The educational management of adolescents may require additional procedures, such as behavioral contracting. This approach involves a teacher and child signing a formal, written, dated contract listing the duties and obligations of the child as well as the privileges or rewards that the teacher will supply.

Studies have shown classroom behavior management programs to be effective for improving classroom behavior as well as compliance at home. However, the children studied did not usually attain normal levels of functioning. This approach was generally less effective than stimulant treatment, and long-term changes and generalization to other situations have yet to be demonstrated.[224]

One reason for poor results of some school interventions is the tendency to overlook the crucial role of academic instruction matched to the ADHD student's ability.[79] Children with ADHD often have learning disabilities; consequently, they have difficulty in reading, writing, spelling, or math. Attention problems and impulsivity in early grades may lead to learning gaps that create further frustration and disruptive behavior.

Academic Skills Therapy

Children with ADHD demonstrate impaired school performance on a number of levels. As a result, programs for teaching academic skills need to target both specific and general skills. Academic skills are generally taught in special classes or by individual tutors using cognitive-behavioral strategies. Peer tutoring (see page 66) can provide more immediate feedback frequency for children with ADHD.

To date, little research has been conducted in the area of academic skills therapy; however, preliminary results of individual case studies are promising, and comprehensive reviews show that specific classroom accommodations help both students and teachers.[225] A meta-analysis of 62 studies found that contingency management strategies coupled with academic interventions were more effective for behavior change than cognitive-behavioral strategies (e.g., self-talk or problem solving) alone.[219]

Social Skills Therapy

Social skills therapy is based on evidence that social interactions play an important role in ADHD. For instance, children who do not know how to wait their turn or compromise are likely to be rejected when playing with others. This rejection can lead to anger or depression, which may be acted on inappropriately by fighting or withdrawal, making the problem worse. When children repeatedly fail in social settings, they may also develop negative associations with schoolwork or getting along with peers. Social skills therapy combines a variety of methods, including:[226]

> **Interaction skills** — Building skills necessary for positive social interactions, such as:
>> ■ Making an introduction to someone new
>> ■ "Asking" rather than "telling"
>> ■ Making a request of a teacher
>> ■ Asking peers to join a game

Clinicians should address both classroom behavioral problems and instruction level.

Specific skills taught might include reading, math, or spelling. General skills training should include:
- ▶ *Organization skills*
- ▶ *Study skills*
- ▶ *Note-taking*
- ▶ *Self-monitoring of behavior and errors*

▶ **Problem solving** — Developing solutions to problems typical for the age group presented, then modeling and rehearsing those solutions. Specific activities include:

■ Listing probable outcomes or consequences for the varying solutions to a problem

■ Determining pros and cons for each solution

■ Listing how each solution affects other people

■ Rehearsing and refining the chosen solutions

▶ **Conflict resolution** — Teaching basic and appropriate communication skills that allow children to state their viewpoint and clearly make requests. In addition, this approach helps teach children how to share, wait, take turns, and control impulsiveness.

The teacher can have a child practice specific impulse control strategies, (e.g., counting to 10 or taking three breaths) and cognitive rehearsal strategies (e.g., saying to themselves, "I can wait," or "It will be my turn soon.")

Therapy also focuses on controlling aggressive behaviors by altering hostile interpretations of events and increasing appropriate coping skills. For instance, if the patient waiting in a line suddenly gets pushed from behind, social skills therapy would involve identifying possible reasons for this event, such as, "The other person tripped," or "She was not paying attention." Then the patient would decide on an appropriate response, such as talking to the person, talking to the teacher, or ignoring the shove.

▶ **Anger management** — Teaching children how to cope with provocations that typically elicit anger and aggression. Once patients identify these situations, they can discuss thoughts that increase the anger ("hot thoughts") as well as alternative thoughts less likely to produce anger ("cool thoughts"). For example, an adolescent may say, "I get angry when I can't go out with my friends." Hot thoughts associated with this situation might be, "I never get to do anything." A cool thought might be, "I don't get to do what I want sometimes, and I don't like it."

Other anger management strategies include:

▶ *Leaving the situation before blowing up*

▶ *Asking a friend or teacher for help*

▶ *Writing an angry letter that doesn't get mailed*

▶ *Engaging in regular physical activity to release built-up energy*

The results of social skills therapy have been mixed. Some studies have noted short-term changes or positive results evident to teachers and parents, but not to peers. One study of inpatients with ADHD involved teaching social-cognitive skills in a group setting as well as providing feedback and reinforcement throughout the day. This study reported patients having increased social skills and reduced loneliness at a one-year follow-up.[227] Some cognitive-behavioral programs for anger control outperform medication in terms of enhanced self-control, decreased physical retaliation, and use of positive coping strategies.[228]

However, evidence generally suggests that, as with other behavioral therapies, the success of social skills therapy often depends on the situations in which it is taught. For example, great gains in social skills can be seen in a therapy group, but vanish in other settings. One promising way around this problem is teaching these skills in broader contexts. For example, one study found this approach effective when used by trained student-mediators, who intervened in conflicts on the playground, and then immediately engaged the participants in problem-solving tactics.[229] Others have suggested including social skills therapy as part of parent training to increase the effectiveness.

Other Traditional Psychotherapeutic Approaches and ADHD

Data from the MTA study (see appendix C) shows that the outcomes of all treatment modalities — medication, psychosocial therapy, and combined therapy — improved ADHD symptoms and decreased the level of negative and ineffective parental discipline.[230, 231] Other traditional psychotherapies besides cognitive-behavioral ones can be useful for some patients.

Children with coexisting anxiety disorders, particularly those with overlapping disruptive disorder, benefit from behavioral and combined interventions.[210]

The Family Therapy Approach to Treating ADHD

Because of the inattention and overactivity of the child with ADHD, family therapy is most successful when it includes psychoeducational techniques. These techniques involve frequent practice and skill rehearsal and may include parent training and problem-solving. Barkley developed an extensive program utilizing cognitive-behavioral techniques combined with a family systems approach. His program includes family and parent sessions as well as a children's group.[108]

The Psychodynamic/Developmental Therapy Approach to Treating ADHD

At best, some psychodynamic/development theories address the interaction of personality, biology, and environmental pressures on ADHD. For instance, parents dealing with sleeping or feeding difficulties with their child may spend excessive amounts of time and become extremely frustrated completing basic care taking tasks. This limits the time parents have for positive play with their child. As a result, parents may feel angry, guilty, and helpless, while the child becomes increasingly agitated or irritable in response. Thus, a pattern of increasingly negative responses can lead to inattention, impulsivity, and hyperactivity.

No developmental or psychodynamic theory provides a comprehensive explanation for ADHD's origin or treatment.

Individual psychodynamic psychotherapy has proven ineffective for treating children diagnosed with ADHD.[232] Some evidence indicates that the reason psychotherapy may be ineffective is that the inattention and over activity characteristic of ADHD precludes the ability to clarify inner thoughts and feelings. However, adults may benefit from certain types of individual therapy that emphasize cognitive and behavioral changes to manage their disorder.

How Effective is a Multimodal Therapy Approach?

Multimodal interventions need to occur early, with long-term treatment and follow-up to address changing needs or problems in relationships, academics, or at home as the individual matures.

Multimodal therapy combines medication and psychosocial treatments. This combination is believed to provide the best treatment possible and is recommended by most clinicians. Multimodal therapy generally includes:

- ▶ Medication therapy
- ▶ Parent training
- ▶ Classroom management
- ▶ Behavioral reinforcement
  (direct contingency management)
- ▶ Social skills therapy

See appendix C for a complete discussion on how the MTA study was structured and specific results.

Past research has found only slight advantages for this approach over the use of medication alone.[233] However, treatments were conducted over relatively short periods of time. To more fully understand which components of multimodal treatment most benefit those with ADHD, the National Institute of Mental Health (NIMH) and the U.S. Department of Education conducted a long-term, well-designed research study — the Multimodal Treatment Study of ADHD (MTA) — that compared psychosocial treatments and medication treatments.

In general, the results of the study validate the use of multimodal therapy and show that extremely well-delivered, multimodal therapy can produce significant advantages over medication or psychosocial treatments alone or standard treatment received in the community.

MTA Follow-up Conclusions for Psychosocial and Medication Therapy with ADHD Children[168]

At the end of 14 months, children were normalized as follows:

- **For medication-treated children,** 82 percent were normalized with only 15 to 18 percent still meeting ADHD criteria.

- **For the psychosocial treatment group and those in the community treatment group who received no medications,** 67 percent were normalized and no longer met ADHD diagnostic criteria.

- **For the combined medication/psychosocial therapy group,** children showed no significant advantage over the medication-only group for inattention, hyperactivity/impulsivity, and oppositional-defiant symptoms. However, **combined medication and psychosocial therapy was superior for symptoms related to anxiety, academic underachievement, and poor social skills** to medication alone or community treatment.[234]

What Psychological Treatments are Used for Treating Adults with ADHD?

Adults seeking treatment for ADHD tend to focus on chronic difficulties that interfere with employment, relationships, or emotional adjustment. Such difficulties include difficulty sustaining attention, forgetfulness, distractibility, impulsive decision making, being hot tempered, inability to complete tasks, and difficulty focusing on a job.

Treatment of adults with ADHD focuses on:

► *Psychoeducation*

► *Coaching*

► *Environmental restructuring*

► *Psychotherapy*

Psychoeducation: Understanding ADHD

Just as children and parents have questions and misconceptions about the disorder, adults with ADHD want to learn about possible causes, symptoms, and treatment. This knowledge helps them feel more control over their lives rather than feeling helpless and frustrated. Some experts believe that educating adults with ADHD about their illness is one of the most important components of successful treatment.[65]

Long-term follow-up studies reveal that many adults with ADHD feel the understanding they gained from an explanation of the disorder was the single most important factor in their ultimate success.[235] Giving patients a clear understanding of what is known about the disorder has the potential to create a profound shift in the patients' self-image and optimism, while giving them the motivation to alter their behavior. Often the realization that they are not stupid, lazy, or bad — appellations they have received all their lives — comes as a profound and positive revelation.

Coaching: Teaching Problem-oriented Skills

The term "coaching" is relatively new. Hallowell proposed 50 tips for managing ADHD by individuals and Hallowell and Ratey developed 25 tips for helping couples.[236, 237] This common-sense approach has spawned Internet coaching, dozens of coaching books. and professional coaching associations.[238] Unfortunately, no controlled evidence demonstrates that these techniques are effective or that they can be maintained by adults with ADHD.

Coaches assist patients by:

► *Helping them to organize their day and work week*

► *Developing time-management skills*

► *Dealing with difficult interpersonal situations*

► *Navigating the activities of daily living*

Environmental Restructuring: Maximizing School and Work Settings

ADHD clinical experience with adults indicates the importance of restructuring patients' environments to improve their life functioning at school, work, and home.[239] Guides available for helping students with ADHD use a variety of useful strategies, including finding appropriate accommodations and fitting the student's educational needs to the college environment.[240, 241]

A variety of "ADHD-friendly jobs" and "ADHD-unfriendly jobs" have been described by Weiss and colleagues.[239] "Friendly jobs" include becoming an inventor or an independent salesperson. In these positions, the individual has:

- ▶ Room for self-directed activity
- ▶ Scheduling freedom
- ▶ Delegating opportunities
- ▶ Loosely structured time and tasks.

"Unfriendly jobs" include becoming a bank teller, pilot, or freelance contractor. In these jobs, the individual has little room for variation from an established structure or so much lack of structure that the risk of failure and dissatisfaction is high.

Psychotherapy: Using Behavioral, Cognitive, and Relaxation Strategies

For adults with ADHD, learning a variety of self-directed behavioral, cognitive, and relaxation strategies can help alleviate the impact of ADHD symptoms.

Using Behavior Management Principles

Many behavior management principles also apply to self reinforcement. For example, patients can reward themselves for completing a project with a special dinner or a fun activity. Or, they might allow themselves to watch the news or a television show only after completing housework. They also might set up a "punishment" by charging themselves or donating a specified amount of money every time they are late to work or an appointment.

Employing Cognitive Strategies

Patients can use cognitive strategies to adjust their work environment by:

▶ *Getting an answering machine and turning off the volume*

▶ *Playing a tape with white noise*

▶ *Wearing headphones*

▶ *Pinning up pictures or quotations for inspiration*

▶ *Making a study carrel*

▶ *Using a Do Not Disturb sign*

▶ *Buying special colored pens, paper, or other supplies to help with organization*

Cognitive strategies can help patients with organizational skills and self-talk. Organizational skills may include:

- ▶ Using a calendar to show assignments or meetings
- ▶ Breaking a task into small steps that take between 15 and 30 minutes
- ▶ Establishing starting, midpoint, and finishing dates for long projects (and setting the finish date ahead of the actual deadline)
- ▶ Adjusting the work environment to minimize distractions and enhance enjoyment

As with children, adults can use self-talk to increase feelings of control and instill a belief that they can accomplish what they want. Self-talk may consist either of positive self-statements (e.g., "Keep trying; you can do it,") or self-directions (e.g., "To complete this big project, first break it into small parts, then start with part 1.") For some patients, developing a list of important self-statements that they carry around on note cards is helpful.

Using Relaxation Techniques

Stress is an important factor with ADHD adults, and many lead a hurried and scattered lifestyle. A number of techniques exist for helping people relax, which may increase concentration and lessen impulsivity. For example, progressive muscle relaxation involves tensing and relaxing different muscle groups. *Meditation* or *yoga* can help increase relaxation and focus. *Imagery* may help a patient visualize accomplishing a task, or reenergizing in a favorite quiet spot.

Effectiveness of Psychological Therapies with Adults

There is some research supporting the usefulness of relaxation techniques with children, but there are no studies on the efficacy of these techniques with adults.[242] Similarly, at this time no controlled research studies exist on using psychological therapies to treat adults with ADHD. Clinical experience suggests, however, that psychotherapy can be useful for helping patients deal with the subjective effects of medication, restructuring some of their characteristic defensive operations, and improving disrupted relationships that have resulted from ADHD symptoms.[243]

meditation — an activity that combines relaxation with focusing one's thoughts

yoga — a system of exercises for attaining bodily or mental control

imagery — the use of mental images

ADHD is a chronic, lifetime disorder, needing some form of treatment across the lifespan.

Key Concepts for Chapter Four

1. Psychological treatments are especially useful for those who fail to respond or only partially respond to medications, experience severe side effects or toxicity, or go through developmental challenges that require new treatment strategies.

2. Benefits of psychological interventions include helping the patient build new skills for social adjustment, overcoming negative behaviors and thoughts, reducing parental/family stress, and for bolstering academic skills.

3. Psychological approaches **most often used to treat children** with ADHD include direct contingency management, parent training, classroom therapy, academic skills therapy, social skills therapy, and family therapy.

4. Psychological approaches **most often used to treat adults** with ADHD include psychoeducation, coaching, environmental restructuring, behavior management, cognitive strategies, and relaxation therapy. These appear to help patients deal with medication compliance issues, restructure defensive responses, and improve relationships disrupted by ADHD symptoms.

5. For milder cases of ADHD, contingency management has proven highly effective for managing behavior in the classroom.

6. Give patients as much education about ADHD as each individual and family can absorb. Education teaches the patient how to self-manage this chronic disorder.

7. Multimodal treatment that combines medication and psychosocial therapy has proven more effective than medication alone for treating ADHD symptoms related to anxiety, academic underachievement, and poor social skills.

8. Tailor the sequence and timing of multimodal treatment (always indicated) to the individual. Particularly for children, multimodal therapy that includes both home and school intervention is essential.

9. Ensure that skill development for parents at home and children in the classroom as well as self-management techniques for adolescents and adults is an integral part of treatment.

Appendix A:
Assessment Measures

I<small>N</small> this appendix, you will find more detailed information on assessment measures used to diagnose ADHD.

Structured Interviews

- ▶ **NIMH Diagnostic Interview Schedule for Children (DISC)**[93] — This interview requires little or no input from the interviewer and can be administered by trained non-professionals. It covers all childhood diagnoses, but is somewhat subject to over-diagnosis. DISC is available in both written and electronic form and is used in many research studies.

- ▶ **Diagnostic Interview for Children and Adolescents (DICA)**[94] — DICA covers all DSM-IV (TR) diagnoses and is user-friendly. It is available in an excellent computerized version.

- ▶ **Schedule for Affective Disorders and Schizophrenia for School-Age Children (Kiddie-SADS)**[95] — This instrument is very thorough and well-researched. It requires clinical expertise and training to administer. Both current and lifetime versions are available.

- ▶ **Connors Adult ADHD Diagnostic Interview for DSM-IV (CAADID)**[96]

Structured Observations

The Child Behavior Checklist-Direct Observation Form (CBCL-DOF) is a standardized measure that gives the clinician:[105]

- ▶ Scores for mean time on tasks, total problems, and symptoms of behavioral mood disturbance
- ▶ *Normative data*
- ▶ A way to assess a broad spectrum of symptoms

Behavior Rating Scales

Parent Ratings

The Conners Parent Rating Scale-Revised (CPRS-R) — CPRS-R comes in a long form of 80 items and 14 subscales, and a short form, containing 27 items and 4 subscales.[70, 244, 245] As in the earlier versions, the items are scored on a four-point scale (0–3) ranging from "not at all" to "very much" as well as on frequency of occurrence. In addition to the main factors covering oppositional, cognitive, hyperactive, anxious, perfectionistic, social, and psychosomatic problems, the long scale includes the DSM-IV symp-

Assessment measures include:
- ▶ *Structured interviews*
- ▶ *Structured observations*
- ▶ *Behavior rating scales*
- ▶ *Neuropsychological tests*

Figure A.1 on page 78 addresses how clinicians can use assessment measures to determine outcomes of treatment interventions. This information is consistent with the process described in chapter two (page 32).

Kiddie-SADS covers most child psychiatric diagnoses and is widely used in research studies.

normative data — statistical or numerical values that are representative of a large group of people and may be used as a basis for comparison of individual cases

Commonly used parent rating scales include:

▶ *Conners Parent Rating Scale-Revised (CPRS-R)*

▶ *Child Behavior Checklist (CBCL)*

▶ *ADHD Rating Scale*

▶ *Home Situations Questionnaire-Revised (HSQ-R)*

tom scales and an empirically derived ADHD Index. The index provides 12 items that maximize identification of ADHD. The CPRS-R also has a "Global Index" (formerly the "Hyperactivity Index"), which is sensitive to changes resulting from treatment such as medication and/or psychosocial interventions.[7] This index is often used before and after a treatment program.

The Child Behavior Checklist (CBCL) — The CBCL contains 138 items scored on two scales: "Social Competence" and "Behavior Problems."[246] Children with ADHD score high in several areas on the behavior problems scale, including hyperactive, aggressive, and delinquent.

Other parent rating measures used less frequently are:

▶ ADHD Rating Scale, a rating of the 18 DSM-IV factors[247]

▶ Home Situations Questionnaire-Revised (HSQ-R), a more specific measure of attention and concentration across different situations[248]

Teacher Ratings

The Conners Teacher Rating Scale-Revised (CTRS-R) — This scale is similar to the CPRS-R and contains a 59-item long form with the same factors (except psychosomatic) as the parent scale (see previous section).[70, 249] It also is available in a 28-item short scale, containing oppositional, hyperactive, cognitive, and ADHD index scales. The 12-item ADHD index scale can quickly screen patients for ADHD and measure responsiveness to treatment.

Research has found that teachers' expectations and repeated uses of the CTRS-R do not appear to hinder the usefulness of the instrument.

The Child Behavior Checklist-Teacher Report Form (CBCL-TRF) — This is a 126-item questionnaire that consists of two scales: "Adaptive Functioning" and "Behavior Problems."[246] Subscales of the behavior problems scale include: anxious. socially withdrawn, unpopular, self destructive, obsessive/compulsive, inattentive, nervous/overactive, and aggressive.An assessment of an adolescent may include ratings from several teachers. A cross-section of situations, including a class or teacher the student rates as best, worst, or average, will provide good comparison scores and information. A new brief scale for separately testing classroom behavior and academic functioning has promising validity in early trials.[249]

The CBCL-TRF successfully discriminates children with ADHD from other children and has significant correlations with observation, the CBCL, and CTRS.[108, 246]

Self Ratings

The Child Behavior Checklist-Youth Self Report (CBCL-YSR) — This was designed for children and adolescents 11 to 18 years of age.[250] Similar to the teacher and parent forms, scores are rated on competence and behavior problems scales.

The CBCL-YSR is used primarily as a screening tool for symptoms associated with ADHD as there is no definitive category for attentional or hyperactive problems within the instrument.

The Wender Utah Rating Scale (WURS) — This scale was developed for retrospective diagnosis of ADHD in adults.[65] This scale contains 61 items and allows adult patients to rate their own childhood behaviors as descriptive or not descriptive on a five-point scale (0–4). The scale appears to discriminate between adults with ADHD versus a depressed or "normal" population.

Conners/Wells Adolescent Self-Report of Symptoms (CASS) — CASS covers six areas of functioning including cognitive problems, anger control, hyperactivity, family problems, and emotional problems.[36] It is highly effective in discriminating adolescents with ADHD from others.

Conners Adult Attention-Deficit Rating Scale (CAARS) — CAARS is a 42-item scale covering similar factors in adults.[35, 63] Both the CASS and the CAARS include key items for detecting depression and anxiety.

Neuropsychological Tests

The Continuous Performance Task (CPT) — CPT takes about 14 minutes to complete and can be administered from a laptop computer at school or in an office environment.[114] CPT measures response to a certain target stimulus when multiple stimuli are presented rapidly. Scores reflect numbers of correct responses, incorrect responses, and lack of responses. Theoretically, all three scoring factors of the CPT measure sustained attention, while errors of commission also measure impulsivity.

The Freedom from Distractibility (FD) — This factor on the Wechsler Intelligence Scale for Children, third edition, (WISC-III) uses the scores on the "Arithmetic," "Digit Span," and "Coding" subtests to measure attention and distractibility in children.[115] However, FD offers limited usefulness as an ADHD diagnostic tool because its scales are unable to pinpoint what causes a particular score. For example, these scales also measure short-term memory, numeric ability, visual-spatial skills, and perceptual-motor speed.

The Wechsler Adult Intelligence Scale (WAIS) — WAIS has a similar factor. No research has been completed with an adult population, but similar problems exist with the WAIS as with the WISC.

The Matching Familiar Figures Test (MFFT) — MFFT was originally designed to measure impulsivity.[116] Results for the MFFT have been mixed, and success in discriminating ADHD from other disorders has been limited. Also, the MFFT has been inconsistent in detecting changes due to medication.

Other Tests — Because impairments in the functioning of the frontal lobe are thought to be related to ADHD, a variety of other tests have been used, including the Stroop Word-Color Association Test, the Wisconsin Card Sort Test, and a test of working memory.[117, 118] Experts disagree about the usefulness of these measures, despite growing evidence that frontal lobe functions are involved in ADHD. However, these techniques may be particularly useful in difficult diagnostic cases.[256, 257]

Adults with borderline personality disorder or atypical depression seem to score high on the WURS because these groups can have overlapping symptoms.

If CAARS results show higher scores on depression and anxiety items, then more detailed, specific instruments can be used, including:

► *Children's Depression Inventory[251]*

► *Reynolds Adolescent Depression Scale[252]*

► *Beck Depression Inventory (ages 13 to adult)[253]*

The CPT provides one of the few direct measures of attention and impulsivity without reliance on observer ratings alone.[254]

The MFFT derives its scores from response time and total errors in matching pictures to a sample.

Results from objective tests of attention, such as CPT, Wisconsin Card Sort, and Stroop Word-Color Test, are more impaired in adults with ADHD than those without ADHD, though by themselves these tests are too inaccurate for diagnosis.[255]

Figure A.1   Measuring Effects of Treatment Interventions

Target Behavior	Measure	Comment
Hyperactive-Impulsive Behavior, Cognitive Problems, Oppositionality and Conduct Problems, Anxiety, Perfectionism, Psychosomatic Behavior	Revised Conners' Parent and Teacher Rating Scales (Long or Short Forms)[70]	These scales have been carefully developed to cover ADHD symptoms and the most common, co-existing conditions. These longer scales are useful for the beginning and end of medication treatment or for treatment follow-up and re-evaluation.
Key ADHD Symptoms	ADHD Index or Global Index[244]	The 12-item ADHD Index most clearly differentiates patients diagnosed with ADHD from others. The Global Index is a 10-item, composite scale known to be highly medication-sensitive in many studies. These are particularly useful when repeated measurements are needed.
DSM-IV ADHD Symptoms	DSM-IV Subscales in CTRS-R or CPRS-R[245, 249]	These new scales provide norms for the DSM-IV ADHD symptoms on several thousand 6- to 12-year-old children. The adolescent and adult scales include the DSM-IV items as a four-point Likert scale without norms. Teachers and parents can be instructed to administer the scales to cover specific time periods.
Sustained Attention and Impulsivity	Continuous Performance Task (CPT)[114]	This is a 15-minute performance measure in which the child responds to rapidly presented stimuli. It is sensitive to impulsive responding as well as to errors of omission. See page 77 for a more detailed description.
Time on Task	Percent of 15-second intervals in a five-minute period during which the child is actually working on an assignment[104]	This measure is quite treatment-sensitive and differentiates hyperactive from normal children. It requires a trained observer and a means of cueing time intervals. While highly valid, it requires training and personnel and may be most appropriate in treatment studies or controlled trials.
Curriculum-based Learning	Number of words correctly read, spelled, or written in a three-minute period; number of correct responses in three minutes of solving arithmetic problems[258]	Materials are chosen from age- and grade-appropriate levels for the child. These measures are particularly useful in monitoring medication treatment over the course of an academic year. For time-action curves during a day, arithmetic and handwriting are particularly sensitive and can be re-administered with little practice effect and with low subject or examiner burden.
Working Memory	Digits Backwards in One Minute	The digits-backwards test from the Wechsler Intelligence Scale for Children is thought to require close attention and working memory. However, more complicated tests of working memory can be used.[119]
Activity Level	• Actigraph • Grid Crossings	• A small device worn on the wrist or body that measures movements.[259] • A room is divided into grids with tape or electronic sensors. The number of grid crossings is measured in a given time frame.

Appendix B:
Differential Diagnosis

Psychiatric Disorders

Key mental disorders that must be differentiated from ADHD include:

- Anxiety disorders
- Bipolar disorder
- Borderline personality disorder
- Conduct disorder/oppositional defiant disorder/ antisocial personality disorder
- Dysthymia and depression
- Learning disabilities
- Post-traumatic stress disorder
- Schizophrenia
- Histrionic personality disorder
- Substance abuse
- Intermittent explosive disorder

Anxiety Disorders

Researchers estimate that there is a 25 percent overlap between ADHD and anxiety disorders.[260] Common symptoms of anxiety disorders, such as restlessness, irritability, impatience, and sleep disturbance, are similar to those experienced with ADHD. However, signs of impulsivity are not usually reported with anxiety disorders. In addition, anxiety disorder symptoms are generally of shorter duration, are accompanied by signs of autonomic nervous system arousal (e.g., sweaty palms, heart palpitations, dizziness, and frequent urination), and include rumination about the future or potential misfortune.

Anxiety disorders include: overanxious disorder, phobic disorders, generalized anxiety disorder, and post-traumatic stress disorder.

In a treatment setting, individuals with coexisting ADHD and anxiety disorders may be less likely to respond to stimulant medication such as Ritalin.® [261]

Bipolar Disorder

Symptoms of bipolar disorder in children are hard to differentiate from those of ADHD. However, those with bipolar disorder experience more cyclical mood disturbance and more intense hyperactivity and impulsivity than those with ADHD. Tantrums are more extreme and last longer; destructiveness is more purposeful than accidental.

Children with bipolar disorder will anticipate and relish fights rather than just "stumble into them." Biological disturbances will also be exacerbated with bipolar disorder. For example, sleep is minimal and appetite may vary from nonexistent to binge eating. In addition, perceptual disturbances such as *delusions* may occur.

delusions — beliefs that someone maintains despite much evidence to the contrary (e.g., children believing that they are cartoon characters; adults believing that they are superhuman)

Children with mania have significantly higher rates of depression, psychosis, anxiety disorder, conduct disorders, and impaired psychosocial functioning than children with ADHD.[262]

euphoria — a state of extreme elation and heightened activity

Because evidence exists that there is a high rate of ADHD symptoms in adolescents with bipolar disorder, differential diagnosis is critical with this age group. Differentiating between ADHD and bipolar disorder in adolescents and adults relies on an analysis of symptom length and severity. Children with bipolar disorder usually do not experience concrete episodes of depression or mania, but they may exhibit some symptoms in an erratic pattern. Adolescents and adults with bipolar disorder usually have more clearly defined instances of depression and mania, such as sleep disturbance, sudden onset, or delusional symptoms.

Hypomania, a component of bipolar illness, shares many symptoms with ADHD, such as irritability, rapid speech, disrupted sleep, and disorganization. Important differences relate to mood and insight. Individuals with hypomania will demonstrate inappropriate levels of *euphoria* or happiness and deny problems or symptoms.

Borderline Personality Disorder

Important differences exist between borderline personality disorder (BPD) and ADHD, even though impulsivity, substance abuse, and impaired relationships are common to both disorders. With BPD, suicide and self-mutilation are more common, and the symptoms of hyperactivity and inattention are not marked. Though adult relationships for those with ADHD are often impaired or unsuccessful, they are not characterized by intense, wildly fluctuating emotions as with BPD. However, there is some overlap between these disorders, particularly in males.[263, 264]

Conduct Disorder/Oppositional Defiant Disorder/ Antisocial Personality Disorder

Aggressive and antisocial behaviors typical of conduct disorder (CD), oppositional defiant disorder (ODD), and antisocial personality disorder (APD) overlap with behaviors characteristic of ADHD.

Conduct Disorder — In recent research, approximately 30 to 50 percent of those studied exhibited symptoms of both ADHD and CD.[265] People with CD characteristically perform more frequent and more severe acts of physical aggression and illegal acts than those with ADHD. Children and adolescents with CD exhibit more severe and persistent overt hostility than those with ADHD.

Oppositional Defiant Disorder — Those with ODD typically resist doing tasks because they are unwilling to conform to others' demands rather than as a result of inattention and impulsivity. This difference is especially clear when evaluating how those who suffer from each disorder respond to activities in which they are interested. When intrigued, those with ADHD will complete tasks willingly as opposed to those with ODD, who generally will not.

Antisocial Personality Disorder — This disorder has been reported more in adults with ADHD. Researchers estimate that adults with ADHD are about 10 times more likely to have APD.[38] These high rates of co-existence typically result from undiagnosed CD as well as the association of school failure and low work status with both ADHD and APD. APD can be differentiated from ADHD by behaviors that reflect a disregard for others, such as breaking the law, financial irresponsibility, "conning" others for pleasure or profit, and a lack of remorse after hurting someone.

Dysthymia and Depression

Loss of interest and pleasure in normal activities, poor self-esteem, and hopelessness are symptoms of depression. While these symptoms can be the result of ADHD, they can also be independent indicators of dysthymia or major depressive disorder. Recent evidence suggests that there may be a high degree of shared genetic influence between major depressive disorder and ADHD.[266, 267]

Persistent and marked dysphoric mood must be present before a clinician can diagnose a mood disorder. However, the dysphoric mood may be a result of demoralization that has come about from struggling with ADHD. Inattention, irritability, and hyperactivity can result from depression, especially in children. Specific situations may account for some signs of low-level adjustment problems or depression. Recent history of these symptoms without accompanying developmental irregularities would indicate depression rather than ADHD. Depressive symptoms may disappear when ADHD is treated, but if the symptoms are part of an independent depressive disorder, treatment for depression may be needed.

Learning Disabilities

Studies of how often patients experience both ADHD and learning disabilities vary significantly in results, ranging from chance to 30 percent.[265] Because individuals with ADHD usually show some academic difficulty and underachievement, clinicians must determine whether the patient suffers from ADHD, a learning disability, or coexisting disorders. Making a differential diagnosis requires:

▶ Assessment of the degree of impairment and impact on academics

▶ Careful examination of the order in which symptoms appear

When a learning disorder is the primary problem, a patient's disruptive behavior patterns are a response to academic problems. These disruptive behaviors tend to increase with age as the negative experiences that trigger them increase. On the other hand, disruptive behaviors and social problems typical of ADHD will be noticed early and remain consistent over time.

Post-Traumatic Stress Disorder (PTSD)

Research suggests that children with pre-existing ADHD are more vulnerable to PTSD.[268] Because some symptoms of PTSD, such as difficulty concentrating or irritable outbursts, overlap with those of ADHD, clinicians should carefully ascertain whether a child being diagnosed with ADHD has been exposed to a traumatic event that caused intense fear or helplessness, and when the trauma happened in relation to the appearance of ADHD symptoms.

Schizophrenia

The disorganized aspects of schizophrenia, such as speech that quickly changes topic (derailment), disorganized behavior, and inappropriate affect, can be similar to ADHD. However, in schizophrenia these disorganized elements such as inappropriate affect of silliness or laughter are unrelated to the content of the conversation or situation. Additionally, the disorganized behavior tends to be severe enough to impair the ability to perform daily activities, such as bathing, dressing, or preparing meals.

Histrionic Personality Disorder

People with histrionic personality disorder may act like the "class clown" or the "life of the party," or display exaggerated emotion to make themselves the center of attention. Additionally, they may change relationships or jobs frequently, craving new emotional attention. Those with ADHD may also change jobs frequently or have difficulties maintaining friendships; however, this occurs because of disorganization, impulsiveness, or poor attention span. Those who are histrionic are often bored or intolerant of routine because of an inability to delay gratification. Those with ADHD tend to be bored and crave excitement because of a poor ability to sustain attention to the topic at hand.

Substance Abuse Disorders

Those with substance use or withdrawal may exhibit symptoms similar to ADHD, such as irritability, mood swings, hyperactivity, or impaired concentration. Careful evaluation of symptom onset can help differentiate substance abuse from ADHD. ADHD symptoms are pervasive and chronic, while symptoms associated with substance abuse have onset and cessation coordinated with substance use.

Intermittent Explosive Disorder

A failure to resist aggressive impulses resulting in serious injury or destruction of property is the hallmark of intermittent explosive disorder. These behaviors reflect very aggressive impulses as opposed to someone with ADHD, who may engage in destructive behavior because of situational frustration or impulsivity.

Genetic Disorders

Several genetic disorders cause typical ADHD symptoms of inattention and hyperactivity, including:

▶ **Turner syndrome in females** — A disorder resulting from a missing sex chromosome marked by a lack of primary reproductive organs and secondary sexual characteristics (e.g., body hair, body shape, voice tone, and short stature).

▶ **XYY syndrome in males** — A chromosomal abnormality in which a third chromosome is associated with low fertility.

▶ **Fragile X syndrome** — Primarily a male disorder, resulting from dysfunctional development on the X chromosome. Atypical physical features include a long face and large head and ears. Behavioral characteristics include cluttered speech, hyperactivity, autism, and meaningless, repetitive hand movements.

▶ **Neurofibromatosis** — A familial condition afflicting children, characterized by developmental changes in the nervous system, muscles, bones, and skin. Tumors may occur throughout the body in pigmented areas.

▶ **Treated Phenylketonuria (PKU)** — A disease caused by a missing enzyme that results in severe and permanent mental retardation if untreated.

▶ **Pervasive Developmental Disorders (PDD)** — Serious and pervasive dysfunctions of basic psychological functioning in social, cognitive, perceptual, attentional, motor, and/or linguistic functions.

▶ **Autistic Disorder** — A type of PDD marked by the withdrawal from reality into oneself, a tendency to be absorbed in one's thoughts and fantasies.

▶ **Fetal Alcohol Syndrome** — Caused by severe maternal alcoholism during pregnancy, this disease results in abnormal anatomical features and psychological deficits, (e.g., growth deficiencies, skeletal malformations, mental retardation, hyperactivity, and heart murmurs).

Medical Disorders

Each of the following medical disorders has some symptoms similar to ADHD symptoms. A thorough medical evaluation to rule out these disorders is recommended:

- ▶ Head injury
- ▶ Dementia
- ▶ Delirium
- ▶ Tumors: frontal, parietal, and temporal
- ▶ Tourette's disorder
- ▶ Stroke
- ▶ Hyperthyroidism
- ▶ Hypothyroidism
- ▶ Renal insufficiency
- ▶ Hepatic insufficiency
- ▶ Anoxic encephalopathy
- ▶ Vitamin deficiency states
- ▶ Chronic obstructive pulmonary disease
- ▶ Multiple sclerosis
- ▶ Seizures/epilepsy
- ▶ Sensory deficits (e.g., hearing loss)
- ▶ Medication side effects
- ▶ Neurological disorders of vigilance

Appendix C:
The MTA Multimodal Treatment Study

A HALLMARK research study, conducted cooperatively by the National Institute of Mental Health (NIMH) and the U.S. Department of Education, examined which components of pharmacological and psychosocial treatments most benefited patients with ADHD. This study compared:[269]

1. Optimally managed medication treatment vs. intensive psychosocial treatment

2. The additive/synergistic effects of combined medication and psychosocial treatment compared to either treatment delivered alone

3. The relative effectiveness of such systematic treatments delivered by specifically trained clinicians following treatment manuals vs. standard treatment received in the community

Study Design

Patients were randomly assigned to one of four treatment groups based on those receiving:

▶ Medications only

▶ Psychosocial treatment only

▶ Combined medications and psychosocial treatment

▶ Standard treatment in the community of their own choosing (which sometimes involved medication at the discretion of the community physician)

The medications-only treatment group received a careful dosing of methylphenidate (Ritalin®) to an optimal level, based on a detailed treatment manual and management by a skilled pharmacotherapist.

Researchers changed medications only after a clear lack of improvement or in the case of intolerable side effects.

The psychosocial treatment was an intense, multicomponent treatment, using most of the proven individual behavioral and cognitive treatments, including:

▶ Parent training delivered over 14 months in 27 group sessions and eight individual sessions

▶ School intervention involving an assistant to the patient's teacher (a paraprofessional), who received intensive training in behavior-management skills, and parents involved with the teachers after completing several parent-training sessions.

▶ A summer treatment program involving intensive interventions over eight weeks, focusing on peer relationships, compliance with adult requests, classroom skills, and competencies in sports and academic skills.[270]

Training methods included reward, response cost, time out, social skills training, group problem-solving, a "buddy system," daily report card, computer classroom, and individualized behavioral programming.

Study Results

*There was **NO** difference between medication and psychosocial treatment in their effects on anxiety as rated by parents. Neither treatment showed any effects on children's' self-ratings of anxiety.*

In the MTA study, treatments were conducted over 14 months. Specific results include:[234, 271, 272]

1. **For the medication treatment group,** 82 percent of patients were normalized and only 15 to 18 percent still met ADHD diagnostic criteria at the end of the 14-month treatment. When compared to the other treatment groups, the results from administering medications were superior to psychosocial treatment and community treatment on measures of **(basis of ratings shown in parentheses for all results)**:

   ▶ **Inattention** (teachers, parents)

   ▶ **Hyperactivity-impulsivity** (teachers, parents)

   ▶ **Disruptive behavior, interference, and aggression** (direct classroom observations)

*These results indicate that some children may respond equally to psychosocial treatments and medications **received in standard community treatment.***

2. **For the psychosocial treatment group,** 67 percent were normalized and no longer met ADHD diagnostic criteria at the end of the treatment period. Psychosocial therapy was not superior to medication for any of the measures. However, the two treatments equally impacted social skills (especially quarreling and prosocial behavior at home) as assessed by both parents and teachers.

   Psychosocial treatment was superior to standard treatment in the community for hyperactive-impulsive behaviors as rated by teachers. Additionally, psychosocial treatment was equally as effective as standard treatment in the community (including those receiving medications) for:

   ▶ **Inattention** (teachers, parents)

   ▶ **Hyperactive-impulsive behavior** (parents)

   ▶ **Aggression** (teachers, parents)

   ▶ **Anxiety** (parents)

   ▶ **Social skills** (parents)

MTA results indicate that both medications and psychosocial therapies are useful treatments for ADHD when delivered by clinicians using a carefully documented treatment manual.

3. **For the combined treatment group,** results indicated that this approach superior to either treatment alone or to standard community treatment for:

   ▶ **Anxiety** (parents)

   ▶ **Social skills** at home and school (parents)

   ▶ **Academic achievement**

An important point to keep in mind when interpreting these findings is that, although psychosocial treatment seemed to add little to the effects of medication alone for many measures, **it was still highly effective by itself:**

▶ Over 75 percent of the patients in the psychosocial treatment group were successfully maintained without medication throughout the study

▶ By the end of 14 months, over 67 percent of those receiving psychosocial treatment no longer met ADHD diagnostic criteria.

Thus, while the results from combining treatments seldom differed from results of using medication alone, psychosocial treatment alone (as delivered in this study) produced highly significant gains in many areas.

4. **For those receiving standard treatment in the community,** results were inferior to receiving medication alone or receiving combined psychosocial therapy and medication. However, these results were equal in effectiveness to psychosocial treatments for most of the measures.

All study treatments delivered by trained professionals using training manuals were superior in virtually all measures, compared to standard treatment received in the community.

MTA Follow-up Conclusions

Over a 24-month period, researchers collected information on treatment outcome. Follow-up conclusions indicate that:[168]

▶ **Stimulant treatment often improves social functioning, but rarely to normal levels.** Behavioral approaches that combine cognitive and behavioral techniques, targeted directly to children (clinical behavior therapy), with reinforcers managed by parents, teachers, or other adults and peers, have greater promise.

The progress in treating social problems can be attributed to an increase in generalization across settings and an increase in the durability of effects.[273]

▶ **Medication and behavioral treatment may complement each other when used together** — While very effective in the short-run, the biggest drawback of psychosocial therapies is the treatment's failure to generalize across settings and time.

▶ **Effects of behavioral therapy may persist longer than medications once treatment ended, particularly when refreshed by relatively frequent school and home contact.** In the MTA study, behavioral effects continued to improve after being gradually faded out and re-examined 14 months after therapy initiation.[274]

▶ **When overall impact of treatment is assessed with a *composite measure*, then there is a statistical advantage for the combined treatment over medication alone.**[275] Behavioral treatment alone, medical treatment alone, and combined therapy produced

composite measure — a measure constructed using several alternate measures of the same phenomena

significantly greater decreases in a parent-rated measure of negative parenting — negative/ineffective discipline — than did standard community treatment.[214] Overall, the success of combination treatment for important school-related outcomes appeared related to reductions in negative and ineffective parenting practices at home.[276]

▶ **Medication algorithms used in the MTA provide effective methods for individual titration of the best medication dose for each patient.**[195] The MTA titration protocol validated the efficacy of weekend methylphenidate (MPH) dosing and established a total daily dose limit of 35 mg of MPH for children weighing less than 25 kg. It replicated previously reported MPH response rates (77 percent), distribution of best doses (10–50 mg/day) across subjects, effect sizes on impairment and deportment as well as dose-related adverse events.[194]

▶ **The nature of a child's comorbid disorders appears to affect which treatments are most beneficial.** Results suggest that there may be three, distinct subtypes of ADHD, depending on comorbid ADHD, ODD, and CD as well as their combinations.[277] In addition, comorbid anxiety disorders impact treatment effectiveness. Outcomes of the MTA study indicate the following:

Despite earlier studies, there was no adverse effect of phobic anxiety on medication response for core ADHD or other outcomes in anxious or non-anxious children with ADHD.[278]

■ Children with parent-defined comorbid anxiety disorders seemed to benefit more from behavior therapy and combined interventions.[277] Analyses of comorbidity moderators showed that children with ADHD and anxiety disorders, particularly those with overlapping disruptive disorder comorbidities (but no ODD/CD) were likely to respond equally well to the MTA behavioral and medication treatments.

■ Children with ADHD only or ADHD with ODD/CD (but without anxiety disorders) responded best to MTA medication treatments (with or without behavioral treatments), while children with multiple comorbid disorders (anxiety and ODD/CD) responded optimally to combined (medication and behavioral) treatments.

▶ **Certain child and family characteristics can moderate treatment response.** Of nine baseline child and family characteristics, none **predicted** treatment outcome, but three **moderated** treatment response. In medication management and combined treatments, parental depressive symptoms and severity of ADHD symptoms in the child were associated with decreased rates of excellent response. When these two characteristics were present, below-average child IQ was an additional moderator.[279]

Glossary

A

affective lability — marked and rapid mood shifts

algorithms — rule-based systems for making decisions

B

behavioral impulsivity — calling out in class, fidgeting, and repeatedly leaving one's seat or getting up "just to check something"

benign — mild, harmless

C

cognitive impulsivity — making frequent mistakes, being disorganized, and producing sloppy work

comorbid — the simultaneous presence of two or more disorders

composite measure — a measure constructed using several alternate measures of the same phenomena

D

deficits in executive functioning — poorly developed skills in areas such as organization, future planning, and project completion

delusions — beliefs that someone maintains despite much evidence to the contrary (e.g., children believing that they are cartoon characters; adults believing that they are superhuman)

distractibility — stimuli in the environment attracts attention away from the task at hand

dopamine and norepinephrine — chemicals in the brain that help regulate motor-control systems and central nervous system functioning

DSM-IV(TR) — the leading diagnostic guide for mental disorders (**Diagnostic and Statistical Manual of Mental Disorders, Fourth Edition, Text Revision**, published by the American Psychiatric Association)

E

euphoria — a state of extreme elation and heightened activity

G

genetic transmission — the transmission of chromosomal links, which influence the development of an organism from one generation to another

I

imagery — the use of mental images

impulsivity/hyperactivity — acting without thinking, often putting the person at risk

inattention — brief attention focus that is often frustrating to others

inhibition — a response caused by specific neurotransmitters binding to receptors on a neuron that decreases the probability that neurotransmitters will be released by the neuron

M

maladaptive behavior — behavior that leads to excessive distress, typically requiring therapy

maternal psychopathology — mental and/or behavioral disorders of the mother

mediating factors — factors that affect the outcome of the trial that is underway

meditation — an activity that combines relaxation with focusing one's thoughts

moderating factors — features at baseline that affect outcome

motor deficits — underdeveloped motor movements and coordination based on expectations by age

multi-method approach — a treatment approach that uses observer ratings, interview, and testing both in clinical medication trials and in individual patient treatment

N

negative self-esteem — overall negative beliefs and feelings people have about themselves

neocortex — the most recently developed and neurologically complex part of the brain

normative data — statistical or numerical values that are representative of a large group of people and may be used as a basis for comparison of individual cases

normed rating scales — assessment tools, validated against a normal population, that measure symptom severity at different developmental periods, such as childhood, adolescence, and adulthood

O

oppositional-defiant behavior — angry, argumentative, resentful, spiteful, and/or vindictive behaviors

P

parasympathetic nervous system — part of the autonomic nervous system that involves restful state bodily functions such as food digestion

peer tutoring — having another student work one-on-one with the student with ADHD

pharmacodynamics — the study of drug action in the body over a period of time, including the processes of absorption, distribution, localization in the tissues, biotransformation, and excretion

pharmacokinetics — the mathematics of the time course of absorption, distribution, metabolism, and excretion (ADME) of drugs in the body, which aids the clinician's ability to individualize medication therapy

prognosis — outcome in the future

psychosocial therapies — therapies that focus on parenting skills, behavior management, education, and social skills

R

reactivity effects — different behaviors than usual, caused by being watched

reinforcement — any consequence that increases the frequency of the preceding behavior

response cost — a form of punishment in which something important is taken away after an undesired behavior takes place

risk model — conceptualization of a disease based on an accumulation of risks that increases the likelihood of a particular disorder emerging

S

self-talk — a strategy of talking oneself through a problem or task either silently or aloud

SSRIs — (Selective Serotonin Reuptake Inhibitors) medications that slow down the ability of nerve cells to absorb serotonin, a neurotransmitter

standard treatment in the community — treatment initiated by parents and chosen from a list of physicians, psychologists, and other mental health providers not affiliated with the research study

standardized — data collected on a large group and results put in the form of averages by age group and gender

stigmatizing — a mark on one's reputation

sympathetic nervous system — part of the autonomic nervous system that regulates arousal functions, such as dilation of pupils, accelerated heart rate, and adrenaline secretion

T

titration — medication dosage adjustment

toxicity — the level of drug in the body at which point the drug acts as a poison

Y

yoga — a system of exercises for attaining bodily or mental control

References

1. American Psychiatric Association (1994). *Diagnostic and statistical manual of mental disorders* (4th ed.), Washington, DC.

2. Anderson, J.C., Williams, S., McGe, R., and Silva, P.A. (1987). DSM-III disorders in preadolescent children: Prevalence in a large sample from the general population. *Archives of General Psychiatry, 44*, 69-76.

3. Costello, E.J., Costello, A.J., Edelbrock, C., Burns, B.J., Dulcan, M.K., Brent, D., and Janiszewski, S. (1985). DSM-III disorders in pediatric primary care: prevalence and risk factors. *Archives of General Psychiatry, 45,* 1107-1116.

4. Szatmari, P., Offord, D.R. and Boyle, M.H. (1989). Ontario Child Health Study: prevalence of attention deficit disorder with hyperactivity. *Journal of Child Psychology and Psychiatry and Allied Disciplines, 30,* 219-230.

5. Shekim, W.O., Kashani, J., Beck, N., Cantwell, D.P., Martin, J., Rosenberg, J., and Costello, A. (1985). The prevalence of attention deficit disorders in a rural midwestern community sample of nine-year-old children. *Journal of the American Academy of Child Psychiatry, 24,* 765-70.

6. Offord, D.R., Boyle, M.H., Szatmari, P., Rae-Grant, N.I., Links, P.S., Cadman, D.T., Byles, J.A., Crawford, J.W., Blum, H.M., Byrne, C., et al. (1987). Ontario Child Health Study. II. Six-month prevalence of disorder and rates of service utilization. *Archives of General Psychiatry, 44,* 832-6.

7. Angold, A., and Costello, E.J. (1998). Three-month prevalence rates for ADHD in the Great Smoky Mountains Epidemiologic Survey. Personal communication.

8. Arcia, E., and Conners, C.K. (1998). Gender differences in ADHD? [In Process Citation]. *Journal of Developmental and Behavioral Pediatrics, 19,* 77-83.

9. Biederman, J., Faraone, S.V., Spencer, T., Wilens, T., Mick, E., and Lapey, K.A. (1994). Gender differences in a sample of adults with attention deficit hyperactivity disorder. *Psychiatry Research, 53,* 13-29.

10. Jensen, P.S. (2002). ADHD: current concepts on etiology, pathophysiology, and neurobiology. *Child & Adolescent Psychiatric Clinics of North America, 9(3),* 557-72, vii-viii.

11. Pliszka, S.R., Greenhill, L.L., et al. (2000). The Texas children's medication algorithm project: Report of the Texas consensus conference panel on medication treatment of childhood attention-deficit/hyperactivity disorder. Part I. Attention-deficit/hyperactivity disorder. [see comment]. *Journal of the American Academy of Child & Adolescent Psychiatry, 39(7),* 908-19.

12. Conners, C.K., March, J.S., et al. (2001). Treatment of attention-deficit/hyperactivity disorder: Expert consensus guidelines. *Journal of Attention Disorders.* S-128.

13. Greenhill, L., Beyer, D.H., et al. (2002). Guidelines and algorithms for the use of methylphenidate in children with Attention-Deficit/Hyperactivity Disorder. *Journal of Attention Disorders, 6(Suppl. 1),* S89-100.

14. Dulcan, M. (1997). Practice parameters for the assessment and treatment of children, adolescents, and adults with attention-deficit/hyperactivity disorder. American Academy of Child and Adolescent Psychiatry. *Journal of the American Academy of Child & Adolescent Psychiatry, 36(10 Suppl.),* 85S-121S.

15. Conners, C.K. (1999). Clinical use of rating scales in diagnosis and treatment of attention-deficit/hyperactivity disorder. *Pediatric Clinics of North America, 46(5),* 857-70, vi.

16. Ernst, M. and Zametkin, A. (1995). "The interface of genetics, neuroimaging and neurochemistry in attention-deficit disorder," in *Psychopharmacology: The fourth generation of progress.* F.E. Bloom and D.J. Kupfer, Editors, Raven Press: New York. (pp.1643-1652).

17. Zametkin, A.J. (1989). The neurobiology of attention-deficit hyperactivity disorder. A synopsis. *Psychiatric Annals, 19,* 584-586.

18. Zametkin, A.J. and Rapoport, J.L. (1987). Review Article: Neurobiology of Attention Deficit Disorder with Hyperactivity: Where have we come in 50 years? *Journal of the American Academy of Child and Adolescent Psychiatry, 26,* 676-686.

19. Biederman, J., Faraone, S.V., Keenan, K., Knee, D., and Tsuang, M.T. (1990). Family-genetic and psychosocial risk factors in DSM-III: attention deficit disorder. *Journal of the American Academy of Child and Adolescent Psychiatry, 29,* 526-533.

20. Deutsch, C.K., Matthysse, S., Swanson, J.M., and Farkas, L.G. (1990). Genetic latent structure analysis of dysmorphology in attention deficit disorder. *Journal of the American Academy of Child and Adolescent Psychiatry, 29*, 189-194.

21. Gillis, J.J., Gilger, J.W., Pennington, B.F., and DeFries, J.C. (1992). Attention deficit disorder in reading disabled twins: evidence for a genetic etiology. *Journal of Abnormal Child Psychology, 20*, 303-315.

22. Stevenson, J. (1992). Evidence for a genetic etiology in hyperactivity in children. *Behavior Genetics, 22*, 337-44.

23. Boudreault, M. and Thivierge, J. (1986). The impact of temperament in a school setting: an epidemiological study. Special Issue: Canadian Academy of Child Psychiatry: A Canadian perspective. *Canadian Journal of Psychiatry, 31*, 499-504.

24. Weissbluth, M. (1984). Sleep duration, temperament, and Conners' ratings of three-year-old children. *Journal of Developmental and Behavioral Pediatrics, 5*, 120-123.

25. Belmaker, R.H. and Biederman, J. (1994). Genetic markers, temperament, and psychopathology [editorial]. *Biological Psychiatry, 36*, 71-2.

26. Nichols, P., and Chen, T.C. (1981). *Minimal brain dysfunction: A prospective study.* (pp. 336). Hillsdale, NJ: Lawrence Erlbaum Associates.

27. Linnet, K.M., Dalsgaard, S., et al. (2003). Maternal lifestyle factors in pregnancy risk of attention deficit hyperactivity disorder and associated behaviors: review of the current evidence. *American Journal of Psychiatry, 160(6)*, 1028-40.

28. McIntosh, D.E., Mulkins, R.S., and Dean, R.S. (1995). Utilization of maternal perinatal risk indicators in the differential diagnosis of ADHD and UADD children. *International Journal of Neuroscience, 81*, 35-46.

29. Biederman, J., Faraone, S.V., Keenan, K., Benjamin, J., Krifcher, B., Moore, C., Sprich-Buckminster, S., Ugaglia, K., Jellinek, M.S., Steingard, R., et al. (1992). Further evidence for family-genetic risk factors in attention deficit hyperactivity disorder. Patterns of comorbidity in probands and relatives psychiatrically and pediatrically referred samples. *Archives of General Psychiatry, 49*, 728-38.

30. Rutter, M., and Casaer, P. (1991). *Biological risk factors for psychosocial disorders.* New York: Cambridge University Press.

31. Rae-Grant, N., Thomas, B.H., Offord, D.R., and Boyle, M.H. (1989). Risk, protective factors, and the prevalence of behavioral and emotional disorders in children and adolescents. *Journal of the American Academy of Child & Adolescent Psychiatry, 28*, 262-8.

32. Werner, E., Bierman, J., French, F., Simonian, K., Connor, A., Smith, R., and Campbell, M. (1968). Reproductive and environmental casualties: a report on the 10-year follow-up of the children of the Kauai pregnancy study. *Pediatrics, 42(1), 112-127*

33. Werner, E. and Smith, R. (1977). *Kauai's children come of age.* Honolulu: University of Hawaii Press.

34. Conners, C.K., and Erhardt, D. (1998). Attention-deficit hyperactivity disorder in children and adolescents, in *Children and Adolescents: Clinical Formulation and Treatment.* M. Hersen and A. Bellack, Editors. New York: Elsevier Science.

35. Conners, C.K., Erhardt, D., Parker, J.D.A., Sitarenious, G., Epstein, J.N., and Sparrow, E. (1998). *The Conners Adult ADHD Rating Scale (CAARS).* Toronto, Canada: Multi-Health Systems, Inc.

36. Conners, C.K., Wells, K.C., Parker, J.D.A., Sitarenios, G., Diamond, J.M., and Powell, J.W. (in press). A new self-report scale for assessment of adolescent psychopathology: Factor structure, reliability, validity and diagnostic sensitivity. *Journal of Abnormal Child Psychology.*

37. Weiss, G., and Hechtman, L. (1993). *Hyperactive children grown up: ADHD in children, adolescents, and adults.* New York: Guilford.

38. Mannuzza, S., Klein, R.G., Bessler, A., Malloy, P., and LaPadula, M. (1993). Adult outcome of hyperactive boys: Educational achievement, occupational rank, and psychiatric status. *Archives of General Psychiatry, 50*, 565-576.

39. Personal communication from Russell Barkley to C. Keith Conners (1998).

40. Applegate, B., Lahey, B.B., Hart, E.L., Biederman, J., Hynd, G.W., Barkley, R.A., Ollendick, T., Frick, P.J., Greenhill, L., McBurnett, K., et al. (1997). Validity of the age-of-onset criterion for ADHD: a report from the DSM-IV field trials. *Journal of the American Academy of Child & Adolescent Psychiatry, 36*, 1211-21.

41. Rae-Grant, N., Thomas, B.H., et al. (1989). Risk, protective factors, and the prevalence of behavioral and emotional disorders in children and adolescents. *Journal of the American Academy of Child & Adolescent Psychiatry, 28(2)*, 262-8.

42. Beitchman, J.H., Wekerle, C., and Hood, J. (1987). Diagnostic continuity from preschool to middle childhood. *Journal of the American Academy of Child and Adolescent Psychiatry, 26*, 694-699.

43. Gillberg, C., Kadesjo, B. (2003). Why bother about clumsiness? The implications of having developmental coordination disorder (DCD). *Neural Plasticity, 10(1-2)*, 59-68.

44. Breznitz, Z., and Friedman, S.L. (1988). Toddlers' concentration: does maternal depression make a difference? *Journal of Child Psychology & Psychiatry & Allied Disciplines, 29*, 267-79.

45. Campbell, S.B., Breaux, A.M., Ewing, L.J., and Szumowski, E.K. (1984). A one-year follow-up study of parent-referred hyperactive preschool children. *Journal of the American Academy of Child Psychiatry, 23*, 243-249.

46. McGee, R., Partridge, F., Williams, S., and Silva, P.A. (1991). A twelve-year follow-up of preschool hyperactive children. *Journal of the American Academy of Child and Adolescent Psychiatry, 30*, 224-232.

47. Kaplan, B.J., McNicol, J., Conte, R.A. and Moghadam, H.K. (1987). Physical signs and symptoms in preschool-age hyperactive and normal children. *Journal of Developmental and Behavioral Pediatrics, 8*, 305-310.

48. Blackman, J.A. (1999). Attention-deficit/hyperactivity disorder in preschoolers. Does it exist and should we treat it? *Pediatric Clinics of North America, 46(5)*, 1011-25.

49. Conner, D.F. (2002). Preschool attention deficit hyperactivity disorder: a review of prevalence, diagnosis, neurobiolgy, and stimulant treatment. *Journal of Developmental and Behavioral Pediatrics, 23(1 Suppl)*, S1-9.

50. McDonnell, M.A., Glod, C. (2003). Prevalence of psychopathology in preschool-age children. *Journal of Child & Adolescent Psychiatric Nursing, 16(4)*, 141-52.

51. Abikoff, H.B., Jensen, P.S., et al. (2002). Observed classroom behavior of children with ADHD: relationship to gender and comorbidity. *Journal of Abnormal Child Psychology, 30(4)*, 349-59.

52. Arcia, E., and Conners, C.K. (1998). Gender differences in ADHD? *Journal of Developmental & Behavioral Pediatrics, 19(2)*, 77-83.

53. Newcorn, J.H., Halperin, J.M., et al. (2001). Symptom profiles in children with ADHD: effects of comorbidity and gender. *Journal of the American Academy of Child & Adolescent Psychiatry, 40(2)*, 137-46.

54. Milich, R., Landau, S., Kilby, G., and Whitten, P. (1982). Preschool peer perceptions of the behavior of hyperactivity and aggressive children. *Journal of Abnormal Child Psychology, 10*, 497-510.

55. Conners, C.K., Wells, K.C., et al. (1997). A new self-report scale for assessment of adolescent psychopathology: Factor structure, reliability, validity and diagnostic sensitivity. *Journal of Abnormal Child Psychology, 25(6)*, 487-497.

56. Biederman, J., Faraone, S., et al. (1996). Predictors of persistence and remission of ADHD into adolescence: results from a four-year prospective follow-up study. *Journal of the American Academy of Child & Adolescent Psychiatry, 35(3)*, 343-51.

57. Klein, R.G., and Mannuzza, S. (1991). Long-term outcome of hyperactive children: A review. Special section: longitudinal research. *Journal of the American Academy of Child and Adolescent Psychiatry, 30*, 383-387.

58. Murphy, K.R., and Barkley, R.A. (1996). Prevalence of DSM-IV symptoms of ADHD in adult licensed drivers: implications for clinical diagnosis. *Journal of Attention Disorders, 1*, 147-161.

59. Conners, C.K., Erhardt, et al. (1999). Self-ratings of ADHD symptoms in adults: I. Factor and normative data. *Journal of Attention Disorders, 3(3)*, 141-151.

60. Reader, M.J., Harris, E.L., et al. (1994). Attention deficit hyperactivity disorder and executive dysfunction. *Developmental Neuropsychology, 10(4)*, 493-512.

61 Pennington, B.F., Ozonoff, S. (1996). Executive functions and developmental psychopathology. *Journal of Child Psychology & Psychiatry, 37(1)*, 51-87.

62. Barkley, R.A. (1997). Behavioral inhibition, sustained attention, and executive functions: constructing a unifying theory of ADHD. *Psychol Bulletin, 121(1)*, 65-94.

63. Conners, C.K., Erhardt, D., Parker, J.D.A., Sitarenios, G., Epstein, J.N., and Sparrow, E. (submitted). The Conners' Adult ADHD Rating Scale (CAARS): standardization, norms, reliability and validity.

64. Spencer, T., Biederman, J., Wilens, T., and Faraone, S.V. (1994). Is attention-deficit hyperactivity disorder in adults a valid disorder? *Harvard Rev Psychiatry, 1*, 326-335.

65. Wender, P.H. (1995). *Attention-deficit hyperactivity disorder in adults.* Oxford, UK: Oxford University Press.

66. Hallowell, E. and Ratey, J. (1994). *Driven to distraction.* New York: Pantheon.

67. Conners, C.K., Erhardt, D., et al. (1999). Self-ratings of ADHD symptoms in adults: I. Factor structure and normative data. *Journal of Attention Disorders.* 141-151.

68. Handen, B., Janosky, J., and McAuliffe, S. (1997). Long-term follow-up of children with mental retardation/borderline intellectual functioning and ADHD. *Journal of Abnormal Child Psychology, 25*, 287-95.

69. Weiss, M., Hechtman, L., et al. (1999). *ADHD in adulthood: A guide to current theory, diagnosis, and treatment.* Baltimore, Maryland: The Johns Hopkins University Press.

70. Conners, C.K. (1997). *Conners' Rating Scales - Revised: Technical Manual.* North Tonawanda, NY: Multi-Health Systems.

71. Kuhne M., Schachar, R., and Tannock, R. (1997). Impact of comorbid oppositional or conduct problems on attention-deficit hyperactivity disorder. *Journal of the American Academy of Child & Adolescent Psychiatry, 36*, 1715-25.

72. Conners, C.K. (2003). Functional impairments in ADHD: The therapeutic target. *Contemporary Pediatrics, 1*, 4-6.

73. Conners, C.K. (1986). How is a teacher rating scale used in the diagnosis of attention deficit disorder? *Journal of Children in Contemporary Society, 19(1-2)*, 33-52.

74. Conners, C.K., Sitarenios, G., et al. (1998). Revision and restandardization of the Conners Teacher Rating Scale (CTRS-R): factor structure, reliability, and criterion validity. *Journal of Abnormal Child Psychology, 26(4)*, 279-291.

75. Atkins, M.S., Pelham, W.E., and Licht, M.H. (1985). A comparison of objective classroom measures and teacher ratings of attention deficit disorder. *Journal of Abnormal Child Psychology, 13*, 155-167.

76. Hodges, K., Wong, M.M. (1996). Psychometric characteristics of multidimensional measure to assess impairment: The child and Adolescent Functional Assessment Scale. *Journal of Child & Family Studies, 5(4)*, 445-467.

77. Bird, H.R., Shaffer, D., et al. (1993). The Columbia Impairment Scale (CIS): Pilot findings on a measure of global impairment for children and adolescents. *International Journal of Methods in Psychiatric Research, 3*, 167-176.

78. Conners, C.K. (2005). Personal communication. Kansas City, MO: Compact Clinicals.

79. Schulte, A.C., Osborne, S.S., and McKinney, J.D. (1990). Academic outcomes for students with learning disabilities in consultation and resource programs. *Exceptional Children, 57*, 162-172.

80. Rowe, K., and Rowe, K. (1992). The relationship between inattentiveness in the classroom and reading achievement (Part B): An explanatory study. *Journal of the American Academy of Child and Adolescent Psychiatry, 31*, 357-368.

81. Biederman, J., Lapey, K.A., Milberger, S., Faraone, S.V., Reed, E.D., and Seidman, L.J. (1994). Motor preference, major depression and psychosocial dysfunction among children with attention deficit hyperactivity disorder. *Journal of Psychiatric Research, 28*, 171-84.

82. Biederman, J., Faraone, S.V., Keenan, K., Steingard, R., and Tsuang, M.T. (1991). Familial association between attention deficit disorder and anxiety disorders. American Journal of Psychiatry. *American Journal of Psychiatry, 148*, 251-6.

83. Biederman, J., Faraone, S.V., Keenan, K., and Tsuang, M.T. (1991). Evidence of familial association between attention deficit disorder and major affective disorders. *Archives of General Psychiatry, 48*, 633-42.

84. Biederman, J., Rosenbaum, J.F., Bolduc, E.A., Faraone, S.V., and Hirshfeld, D.R. (1991). A high-risk study of young children of parents with panic disorder and agoraphobia with and without comorbid major depression. *Psychiatry Research, 37*, 333-48.

85. Fendrich, M., Weissman, M.M., Warner, V., and Mufson, L. (1990). Two-year recall of lifetime diagnoses in offspring at high and low risk for major depression: The stability of offspring reports. *Archives of General Psychiatry, 47*, 1121-1127.

86. Bowring, M. and Kovacs, M. (1992). Difficulties in diagnosing manic disorders among children and adolescents. *Journal of the American Academy of Child and Adolescent Psychiatry, 31*, 611-614.

87. Conners, C.K. and Sparrow, E. (1998). Nootropics and foods, in *Practitioner's Guide to Psychoactive Drugs for Children and Adolescents (2ⁿᵈ Edition)*, J.S. Werry and M. Aman, Editors. New York: Plenum Press.

88. Conners, C.K. (1984). Nutritional therapy in children, in *Nutrition and Behavior.* J. Galler, Editor. New York: Plenum Press. 159-192.

89. Tuthill, R. (1996). Hair lead levels related to children's classroom attention-deficit behavior. *Archives of Environmental Health, 51*, 214-220.

90. Stewart, P. and Sandra, M. (1989). Attention deficit disorder: A toxic response to ambient cadmium air pollution. *International Journal of Biosocial and Medical Research, 11*, 134-143.

91. Grundfast, K.M., Berkowitz, R.G., Conners, C.K., and Belman, P. (1991). Complete evaluation of the child identified as a poor listener. *International Journal of Pediatric Otorhinolaryngology, 21*, 65-78.

92. Pillsbury, H.C., Grose, J.H., Coleman, W.L., Conners, C.K., and Hall, J.W. (1995). Binaural function in children with attention-deficit hyperactivity disorder. *Archives of Otolaryngol Head Neck Surgery, 121, 1345-50.*

93. Shaffer, D., Schwab-Stone, M., Fisher, P., Cohen, P., Piacentini, J., Davies, M., Conners, C.K., and Regier, D. (1993). The Diagnostic Interview Schedule for Children-Revised Version (DISC-R): 1. Preparation, field testing, interrater reliability, and acceptability. *Journal of the American Academy of Child and Adolescent Psychiatry, 32*, 643-650.

94. Reich, W. Welner, Z., and Herjanic, B. (1997). *DICA-IV: Diagnostic interview for children and adolescents-IV.* Toronto: Multi-Health Systems.

95. Kaufamn, J., Birmaher, B., Brent, D., Rao, U., Flynn, C., Moreci, P., Williamson, D., and Ryan, N. (1997). Schedule for Affective Disorders and Schizophrenia for school-age children — Present and Lifetime version (K-SADS-PL): Initial reliability and validity data. *Journal of the American Academy of Child and Adolescent Psychiatry, 36*, 980-988.

96. Conners, C.K. (2001). *Conners' Adult ADHD Diagnostic Interview for DSM-IV.* North Tonawanda, NY: Multi-Health Systems, Inc.

97. Conners, C. and March, J., (1993). *Developmental History Form for ADHD and Related Disorders.* Toronto: Multi-Health Systems, Inc.

98. Conners, C., Erhardt, D., and Sparrow, E. (1998). *CADDI: A structured interview for ADHD and related disorders.* Toronto: Multi-Health Systems.

99. Cantwell, D.P., & Baker, L. (1985). Psychiatric and learning disorders in children with speech and language disorders: A descriptive analysis. In K.D. Gadow (Ed.), *Advances in Learning and Behavioral Disabilities* t(Vol. 4). Greenwich, CT: JAL.

100. Barkley, R.A., Murphy, K., and Kwasnik, D. (1996). Psychological adjustment and adaptive impairments in young adults with ADHD. *Journal of Attention Disorders, 1*, 41-54.

101. Ward, M.F., Wender, P.H., and Reimherr, F.W. (1993). The Wender Utah Rating Scale: An aid in the retrospective diagnosis of childhood attention deficit hyperactivity disorder. *American Journal of Psychiatry, 150*, 885-890.

102. Wilens, T.E., Spencer, T.J., and Prince, J. (1997). Diagnosing ADD in adults, in *Attention!* (pp. 27-35).

103. Sallee, F. (1995). *Attention Deficit/Hyperactivity Disorder in Adults.* Champaign, IL: Grotelueschen Associates.

104. Abikoff, H., Gittelman, R., and Klein, D.F. (1980). Classroom observation code for hyperactive children: A replication of validity. *Journal of Consulting and Clinical Psychology, 48*, 555-565.

105. Achenbach, T.M. and Edlebrock, C. (1986). *Manual for the Teacher Report Form and the Child Behavior Profile.* Burlington, VT: Universtiy of Vermont Department of Psychiatry.

106. Platzman, K.A., Stoy, M.R., Brown, R.T., and Coles, C.D., et al. (1992). Review of observational methods in attention deficit hyperactivity disorder (ADHD): Implication for diagnosis. *School Psychology Quarterly, 7*, 155-177.

107. Goldstein, S., and Goldstein, M. (1998). *Managing attention deficit hyperactivity disorder in children: a guide for practitioners.* (pp. 876). New York: John Wiley & Sons.

108. Barkley, R.A. (1990). *Attention deficit hyperactivity disorder: a handbook for diagnosis and treatment.* New York: Guilford.

109. DuPaul, G.J., Guevremont, D.C., Barkley, R.A. (1992). Behavioral treatment of attention-deficit hyperactivity disorder in the classroom: The use of the attention training system. *Behavioral Modifications, 16(2)*, 204-25.

110. Conners, C.K., Wells, K.C., Parker, J.D., Sitarenios, G., Diamond, J.M., and Powell, J.W. (1997). A new self-report scale for assessment of adolescent psychopathology: factor structure, reliability, validity and diagnostic sensitivity. *Journal of Abnormal Child Psychology, 25(6)*, 487-97.

111. Achenback, T.M., and Edelbrock, C. (1987). *Manual for the youth self-report and profile.* Burlington, VT: University of Vermont Department of Psychiatry.

112. Conners, C.K., Erhardt, D., Parker, J.D.A., Sitarenious, G., Epstein, J.N., and Sparrow, E. (1999). *The Conners Adult ADHD Rating Scale (CAARS).* Toronto: Multi-Health Systems, Inc.

113. Seidman, L.J., Biederman, J., Faraone, S.V., Weber, W., and Ouellette, C. (1997). Toward defining a neuropsychology of attention deficit-hyperactivity disorder: Performance of children and adolescents from a large clinically referred sample. *Journal of Consulting and Clinical Psychology, 65*, 150-160.

114. Conners, C.K. (1994). *The Conners Continuous Performance Test.* Toronto: Multi-Health Systems, Inc.

115. Wechsler, D. (1991). *The Wechsler Intelligence Scale for Children Revised* (3rd edition). New York: The Psychological Corporation.

116. Kagan, J. (1966). Reflection-impulsivity: The generality and dynamics of conceptual tempo. *Journal of Abnormal Psychology, 71*, 17-254.

117. Lufi, D., Cohen, A., and Parish, P.J. (1990). Identifying attention deficit hyperactive disorder with the WISC-R and the Stroop color and word test. *Psychology in the Schools, 27*, 28-34.

118. Grant, D. and Berg, E. (1948). *The Wisconsin Card Sort Test: Directions for administrations and scoring.* Odessa, FL: Psychological Assessment Resources.

119. Tannock, R., Ickowicz, A., and Schachar, R. (1995). Differential effects of methylphenidate on working memory in ADHD children with and without comorbid anxiety. *Journal of the American Academy of Child and Adolescent Psychiatry, 34*, 886-96.

120. Schopick, D. (1998). *Highly effective approaches to making the Conners' CPT work in your clinical practice.* North Tonawanda, NY: Multi-Health Systems, Inc.

121. Schachar, R.J. and Wachsmuth, R. (1991). Family dysfunction and psychosocial adversity: Comparison of attention deficit disorder, conduct disorder, normal and clinical controls. Special Issue: Childhood disorders in the context of the family. *Canadian Journal of Behavioural Science, 23*, 332-348.

122. Moos, R.H. and Moos, B.S. (1986). *Family Environment Scale.* Palo Alto, CA: Consulting Psychologists.

123. Moos, R.H. and Moos, B.S. (1988). *Life stressors and social resources inventory: preliminary manual.* Palo Alto, CA: Stanford University and VA Medical Centers.

124. Miller, I.W., Bishop, D.S., Epstein, N.B. and Keitner, G.I. (1985). The McMaster Family Assessment Device: Reliability and validity. *Journal of Marital and Family Therapy, 11*, 345-356.

125. Abidin, R.R. (1990). *The Parenting Stress Index.* (3rd Ed.) Charlottesville, VA: Pediatric Psychology Press.

126. Waid, L. J., DE; Anton, R.F. (1998). Attention-deficit hyperactivity disorder and substance abuse, in *Dual diagnosis and treatment: Substance abuse and comorbid medical and psychiatric disorders.* H. R. Kranzler, BJ. (ed). (pp. 393-425). New York, Basel & Hong Kong: Marcel Dekker.

127. Kwasman, A., Tinsley, B.J., and Lepper, H.S. (1995). Pediatricians' knowledge and attitudes concerning diagnosis and treatment of attention deficit and hyperactivity disorders: A national survey approach. *Archive of Pediatric Adolescent Medicine, 149*, 1211-6.

128. Rapoport, J.L., Buchsbaum, M.S., Weingartner, H., Zahn, T.P., Ludlow, C., and Mikkelsen, E.J. (1980). Dextroamphetamine: Its cognitive and behavioral effects in normal and hyperactive boys and normal men. *Archives of General Psychiatry, 37(8)*, 933-943.

129. Sostek, A.J., Buchsbaum, M.S., et al. (1980). Effects of amphetamine on vigilance performance in normal and hyperactive children. *Journal of Abnormal Child Psychology, 8(4)*, 491-500.

130. Greenhill, L.L., Abikoff, H.B., Arnold, L.E., Cantwell, D.P., Conners, C.K., Elliott, G., Hechtman, L., Hinshaw, S.P., Hoza, B., Jensen, P.S., et al. (1996). Medication treatment strategies in the MTA Study: Relevance to clinicians and researchers. *Journal of the American Academy of Child and Adolescent Psychiatry, 35*, 1304-13.

131. Goldstein, M. (1998). Medications for ADHD. S. Goldstein and M. Goldstein, (Eds.), *Managing attention-deficit hyperactivity disorder in children.* (p. 878). New York: John Wiley and Sons, Inc.

132. Pliszka, S.R., Greenhill, L.L., et al., (2000). The Texas children's medication algorithm project: Report of the Texas consensus conference panel on medication treatment of childhood attention-deficit/hyperactivity disorder, part I. *Journal of the American Academy of Child & Adolescent Psychiatry, 39(7)*, 908-919.

133. Conners, C.K., March, J.S., et al. (2001). Treatment of attention-deficit/hyperactivity disorder: Expert consensus guidelines. *Journal of Attention Disorders, 4(Suppl. 1)*, S-128.

134. Anonymous (2002). Dexmethylphenidate — Novartis/Celgene. Focalin, D-MPH, D-methylphenidate hydrochloride, D-methylphenidate, dexmethylphenidate, dexmethylphenidate hydrochloride. *Medications in R&D, 3(4)*, 279-82.

135. Keating, G.M., Figgitt, D.P. (2002). Dexmethylphenidate. *Medications, 62(13)*, 1899-904.

136. Cloninger, C.R. (1988). A unified biosocial theory of personality and its role in the development of anxiety states: A reply to commentaries. *Psychiatric Developments, 6*, 83-120.

137. Quay, H.C. (1997). Inhibition and attention deficit hyperactivity disorder. *Journal of Abnormal Child Psychology, 25*, 7-13.

138. Spencer, T., Biederman, J., Wilens, T., Harding, M., O'Donnell, D., and Griffin, S. (1996). Pharmacotherapy of attention-deficit hyperactivity disorder across the life cycle [see comments]. *Journal of the American Academy of Child and Adolescent Psychiatry, 35*, 409-32.

139. Shaywitz, B.A., Klopper, J.H., and Gordon, J.W. (1978). Methylphenidate in 6-hydroxy-dopamine-treated developing rat pups. *Archives of Neurology, 35*, 463-469.

140. Wilens, T.E., Biederman, et al. (2002). Attention deficit-hyperactivity disorder across the lifespan. *Annual Review of Medicine, 53*, 113-31.

141. Rapport, M.D. and Kelly, K.L. (1991). Psychostimulant effects on learning and cognitive function: Findings and implications for children with attention deficit hyperactivity disorder. *Clinical Psychology Review, 11*, 61-92.

142. Douglas, V.I., Barr, R.G., Amin, K., O'Neill, M.E., et al. (1988). Dosage effects and individual responsivity to methylphenidate in attention deficit disorder. *Journal of Child Psychology and Psychiatry and Allied Disciplines, 29*, 453-475.

143. Solanto, M.V. and Conners, C.K. (1982). A dose-response and time-action analysis of autonomic and behavioral effects of methylphenidate in attention deficit disorder with hyperactivity. *Psychophysiology, 19*, 658-667.

144. Copeland, L., Wolraich, M., et al. (1987). Pediatricians' reported practices in the assessment and treatment of attention deficit disorders. *Journal of Developmental and Behavioral Pediatrics, 8(4)*, 191-197.

145. Wolraich, M.L., Lindgren, S., et al. (1990). Stimulant medication use by primary care physicians in the treatment of attention deficit hyperactivity disorder. *Pediatrics, 86(1)*, 95-101.

146. Conners, C.K. (2002). Forty years of methylphenidate treatment in attention-deficit/hyperactivity disorder. *Journal of Attention Disorders, 6(Suppl. 1)*, S17-30.

147. Wilens, T.E., Spencer, T., et al. (1995). Combined pharmacotherapy: an emerging trend in pediatric psychopharmacology [see comments]. Comment in: *Journal of the American Academy of Child & Adolescent Psychiatry*, 1995, Dec., 34(12): 1558, Comment in: Journal of the American Academy of Child & Adolescent Psychiatry, 1995, Dec., 34(12), 1558-9. *Journal of the American Academy of Child & Adolescent Psychiatry, 34(1)*, 110-2.

148. Prince, J.B., Wilens, T.E., et al. (1996). Clonidine for sleep disturbances associated with attention-deficit hyperactivity disorder: A systematic chart review of 62 cases. *Journal of the American Academy of Child & Adolescent Psychiatry, 35(5)*, 599-605

149. Barkley, R.A. (2003). Does the treatment of attention-deficit/hyperactivity disorder with stimulants contribute to medication use/abuse? A 13-year prospective study. *Pediatrics, 111(No. 1)*, 97-109.

150. Satterfield, J.H. (1995). "Prediction of antisocial behavior in attention-deficit hyperactivity disorder boys from aggression/defiant scores": Reply. *Journal of the American Academy of Child & Adolescent Psychiatry, 34*, 398-400.

151. Klein, R.G., Abikoff, H., Klass, E., Ganeles, D., Seese, L.M., and Pollack, S. (1997). Clinical efficacy of methylphenidate in conduct disorder with and without attention deficit hyperactivity disorder. *Archives of General Psychiatry, 54*, 1073-80.

152. Speltz, M.L., Varley, C.K., Peterson, K., and Beilke, R.L. (1988). Effects of dextroamphetamine and contingency management on a preschooler with ADHD and oppositional defiant disorder. *Journal of the American Academy of Child and Adolescent Psychiatry, 27*, 175-178.

153. Biederman, J., Munir, K., and Knee, D. (1987). Conduct and oppositional disorder in clinically referred children with attention deficit disorder: A controlled family study. *Journal of the American Academy of Child & Adolescent Psychiatry, 26*, 724-7.

154. Carlson, C.L., Pelham, W.E.J., Milich, R., and Dixon, J. (1992). Single and combined effects of methylphenidate and behavior therapy on the classroom performance on children with attention-deficit hyperactivity disorder. *Journal of Abnormal Child Psychology, 20*, 213-232.

155. Pelham, W.E., Vodde, H.M., Murphy, D.A., Greenstein, J. and Vallano, G. (1991). The effects of methylphenidate on ADHD adolescents in recreational, peer group, and classroom settings. *Journal of Clinical Child Psychology, 20*, 293-300.

156. Barkley, R.A., Karlsson, J., Pollard, S., and Murphy, J.V. (1985). Developmental changes in the mother-child interactions of hyperactive boys: Effects of two dose levels of Ritalin. *Journal of Child Psychology and Psychiatry and Allied Disciplines, 26*, 705-715.

157. Barkley, R.A. (1988). The effects of methylphenidate on the interactions of preschool ADHD children with their mothers. *Journal of the American Academy of Child and Adolescent Psychiatry, 27*, 336-341.

158. Hinshaw, S.P., Heller, T., and McHale, J.P. (1992). Covert antisocial behavior in boys with attention-deficit hyperactivity disorder: External validation and effects of methylphenidate. *Journal of Consulting and Clinical Psychology, 60*, 274-281.

159. Whalen, C.K. and Henker, B. (1991). Social impact of stimulant treatment for hyperactive children. *Journal of Learning Disabilities, 24*, 231-241.

160. Walker, M.K., Sprague, R.L., Sleator, E.K., and Ullmann, R.K. (1988). Effects of methylphenidate hydrochloride on the subjective reporting of mood in children with attention deficit disorder. Special Issue: Interface between mental and physical illness. *Issues in Mental Health Nursing, 9*, 373-385.

161. Tannock, R., Schachar, R., and Logan, G. (1995). Methylphenidate and cognitive flexibility: Dissociated dose effects in hyperactive children. *Journal of Abnormal Child Psychology, 23, 235-266*.

162. Parker, J.D.A., Sitarenios, G., et al. (1996) Abbreviated Conners' rating scales revisited: A confirmatory factor analytic study. *Journal of Attention Disorders, 1*, 55-62.

163. Parker, J.D.A., Sitarenios, G., et al. (submitted for publication). Assessment of attention-deficit/hyperactivity disorder: A new index for parent, teacher, and adolescent ratings.

164. Elia, J., Borcherding, B.G., et al. (1991). Methylphenidate and dextroamphetamine treatments of hyperactivity: Are there true nonresponders? *Psychiatry Research, 36(2)*, 141-155.

165. Efron, D., Jarman, F., et al. (1997). Side effects of methylphenidate and dexamphetamine in children with attention deficit hyperactivity disorder: A double-blind, crossover trial. *Pediatrics, 100(4)*, 662-666.

166. Brown, R.T., Borden, K.A., et al. (1988). Patterns of compliance in a treatment program for children with attention deficit disorder. *Journal of Compliance in Health Care, 3(1)*, 23-39.

167. Jerome, L. (1995). Teacher and parent influences on medication compliance. *Journal of Child & Adolescent Psychopharmacology, 5(1)*, 85-86.

168. MTA Cooperative Group. (2004). National Institute of Mental Health Collaborative Multimodal Treatment Study of ADHD Follow-up: 24 month outcomes of treatment strategies for attention-deficit/hyperactivity disorder. *Pediatrics, 113(No. 4)*, 754-761.

169. Weiss, M., Jain, U., et al. (2000). Clinical suggestions for management of stimulant treatment in adolescents. *Canadian Journal of Psychiatry - Revue Canadienne de Psychiatric, 45(8)*, 717-23.

171. Firestone, P. (1982). Factors associated with children's adherence to stimulant medication. *American Journal of Orthopsychiatry, 52*, 447-457.

172. Brown, R.T., Borden, K.A., Wynne, M.E., Spunt, A.L., et al. (1987). Compliance with pharmacological and cognitive treatments for attention deficit disorder. *Journal of the American Academy of Child and Adolescent Psychiatry, 26*, 521-526.

173. Brown, R.T. and Pacini, J.N. (1989). Perceived family functioning, marital status, and depression in parents of boys with attention deficit disorder. *Journal of Learning Disabilities, 22*, 581-587.

174. Pine, D.S., Klein, R.G., et al. (1993). Attention-deficit hyperactivity disorder and comorbid psychosis: a review and two clinical presentations [see comments]. *Journal of Consulting and Clinical Psychology, 54(4)*, 140-5.

175. Opler, L.A., Frank, D.M., et al. (2001). Psychostimulants in the treatment of adults with psychosis and attention deficit disorder. *Annals of the New York Academy of Sciences, 931*, 297-301.

176. Kurlan, R. (2003). Tourette's syndrome: are stimulants safe? *Current Neurology & Neuroscience Reports, 3(4)*, 285-8.

177. Wilens, T.E., Faraone, S.V., et al. (2003). Does stimulant therapy of attention-deficit/hyperactivity disorder beget later substance abuse? A meta-analytic review of the literature. *Pediatrics, 111(No. 1)*, 179-185.

178. Pliszka, S.R. (1989). Effect of anxiety on cognition, behavior, and stimulant response in ADHD. *Journal of the American Academy of Child & Adolescent Psychiatry, 28*, 882-887.

179. Elia, J., Borcherding, B.G., Rapoport, J.L., and Keysor, C.S. (1991). Methylphenidate and dextroamphetamine treatments of hyperactivity: Are there true nonresponders? *Psychiatry Research, 36*, 141-155.

180. Sylvester, C.E., and Kruesi, M.J.P. (1994). Child and adolescent psychopharmacotherapy: progress and pitfalls. *Psychiatric Annals, 24*, 83-90.

181. Wilens, T.E., Biederman, J., et al. (1995). A systematic assessment of tricyclic antidepressants in the treatment of adult attention-deficit hyperactivity disorder. *Journal of Nervous & Mental Disease, 183(1)*, 48-50.

182. Popper, C.W. (1997). Antidepressants in the treatment of attention-deficit/hyperactivity disorder. [Review] [176 refs.] *Journal of Clinical Psychiatry, 14*, 14-29.

183. Barrickman, L.L., Perry, P.J., Allen, A.J., Kuperman, S., Arndt, S.V., Herrmann, K.J., and Schumacher, E. (1995). Bupropion versus methylphenidate in the treatment of attention-deficit hyperactivity disorder. *Journal of American Academy of Child Adolescent Psychiatry, 34*, 649-657.

184. Conners, C.K., Casat, C.D., Gualtieri, C.T., Weller, E., Reader, M., Reiss, A., Weller, R.A., Khayrallah, M., and Ascher, J. (1996). Bupropion hydrochloride in attention deficit disorder with hyperactivity. *Journal of the American Academy of Child & Adolescent Psychiatry, 35*, 1314-1321.

185. Emslie, G.J., Walkup, J.T., et al. (1999). Nontricyclic antidepressants: Current trends in children and adolescents. *Journal of the American Academy of Child & Adolescent Psychiatry, 38(5)*, 517-28.

186. Steingard, R., Biederman, J., et al. (1992). Comparison of clonidine response in the treatment of attention-deficit hyperactivity disorder with and without comorbid tic disorders. *Journal of the American Academy of Child and Adolescent Psychiatry, 32(2)*, 350-353.

187. Walkup, J.T. (1995). Methylphenidate and clonidine. *American Academy of Child and Adolescent Psychiatry News*, Sept-Oct., 11-15.

188. Olvera, R.L., Pliszka, S.R., et al. (1996). An open trial of venlafaxine in the treatment of attention-deficit/hyperactivity disorder in children and adolescents. *Journal of Child & Adolescent Psychopharmacology, 6(4)*, 241-50.

189. Conners, C.K., Levin, E.D., et al. (1996). Nicotine and attention in adult attention deficit hyperactivity disorder (ADHD). *Psychopharmacology Bulletin, 32(1)*, 67-73.

190. Levin, E.D., Conners, C.K., et al. (2001). Effects of chronic nicotine and methylphenidate in adults with attention deficit/hyperactivity disorder. *Experimental & Clinical Psychopharmacology, 9(1)*, 83-90.

191. Mihailescu, S., Drucker-Colin, R. (2000). Nicotine, brain nicotinic receptors, and neuropsychiatric disorders. *Archives of Medical Research, 31(2)*, 131-44.

192. Swanson, J.M., McBurnett, K., Wigal, T., Pfiffner, L., Lerner, M.A., Williams, L., Christian, D.L., Tamm, L., Willcutt, E., Crowley, K., et al. (1995). Effect of stimulant medication on children with attention deficit disorder: A review of reviews. *Exceptional Children, 60*, 154-162.

193. Gillberg, C., Melander, H., von Knorring, A.L., Janols, L.O., Thernlund, G., Hagglof, B., Eidevall-Wallin, L., Gustafsson, P., and Kopp, S. (1997). Long-term stimulant treatment of children with attention deficit hyperactivity disorder symptoms. *Archives of General Psychiatry, 54*, 857-864.

194. Greenhill, L.L., Swanson, J.M., et al. (2001). Impairment and deport responses to different methylphenidate doses in children with ADHD: the MTA tritration trial. *Journal of the American Academy of Child & Adolescent Psychiatry, 40(2)*, 180-7.

195. Greenhill, L.L., Abikoff, H.B., et al. (1996). Medication treatment strategies in the MTA study: Relevance to clinicians and researchers. *Journal of the American Academy of Child and Adolescent Psychiatry, 35(10)*, 1304-13.

196. Maidment, I.D. (2003). Efficacy of stimulants in adult ADHD. *Annals of Pharmacotherapy, 37(12)*, 1884-90.

197. Maidment, I.D. (2003). The use of antidepressants to treat attention deficit hyperactivity disorder in adults. *Journal of Psychopharmacology, 17(3)*, 332-6.

198. Anonymous (1998). *NIH consensus development conference on diagnosis and treatment of attention deficit hyperactivity disorder.* Bethesda, MD: National Institute of Health

199. Goldman, L.S., Genel, et al. (1998). Diagnosis and treatment of attention-deficit/hyperactivity disorder in children and adolescents. Council on Scientific Affairs, American Medical Association. *JAMA, 279(14)*, 1100-7.

200. Greene, R., Biederman, J., et al. (1997). Adolescent outcome of boys with attention-deficit/hyperactivity disorder and social disbility: Results from a 4-year longitudinal follow-up study. *Journal of Consulting & Clinical Psychology, 65(5)*, 758-67.

201. Whalen, C.K. and Henker, B. (1985). The social worlds of hyperactive (ADHD) children. Special Issue: Attention deficit disorder: Issues in assessment and intervention. *Clinical Psychology Review, 5*, 447-478.

202. Cunningham, C.E. and Barkley, R.A. (1978). The effects of methylphenidate on the mother-child interaction of hyperactive identical twins. *Developmental Medicine and Child Neurology, 20*, 634-642.

203. Ricchini, W. (1997). Self-esteem & ADHD: Too important to overlook. *Advance for Nurse Practitioners, 5*, 98116334

204. DuPaul, G., Anastopoulos, A., Kwasnik, D., Barkley, R., and McMurray, M. (1996). Methylphenidate effects on children with attention deficit hyperactivity disorder: Self-report of symptoms, side-effects, and self-esteem. *Journal of Attention Disorders, 1*, 3-15.

205. Abikoff, H., Ganeles, D., et al. (1988). Cognitive training in academically deficient ADHD boys receiving stimulant medication. *Journal of Abnormal Child Psychology, 16(4)*, 411-432.

206. Abikoff, H. (1991). Cognitive training in ADHD children: Less to it than meets the eye. *Journal of Learning Disabilities, 24(4)*, 205-9.

207. Hinshaw, S., March, J., et al. (1997). Comprehensive assessment of childhood attention-deficit hyperactivity disorder in the context of a multisite, multimodal clinical trial. *Journal of Attention Disorders, 1*, 217-234.

208. Schulte, A.C., Osborne, S.S. (1989). *Prevalence estimates and patterns of achievement deficits in an independently selected sample of learning disabled students.* San Francisco, CA: International Council for Exceptional Children.

209. Gadow, K.D. (1985). Relative efficacy of pharmacological, behavioral, and combination treatments for enhancing academic performance. Special Issue: Attention deficit disorder: Issues in assessment and intervention. *Clinical Psychology Review, 5*, 513-533.

210. Jensen, P.S., Hinshaw, S.P., et al. (2001). Findings from the NIMH Multimodal Treatment Study of ADHD (MTA): implications and applications for primary care providers. *Journal of Developmental & Behavioral Pediatrics, 22(1)*, 60-73.

211. Abidin, R.R. (1990). *The Parenting Stress Index.* Charlottesville, VA: Pediatric Psychology Press.

212. Anastopoulos, A.D., Guevremont, D.C., et al. (1992). Parenting stress among families of children with attention deficit hyperactivity disorder. *Journal of Abnormal Child Psychology, 20(5)*, 503-20.

213. Wahler, R.G. and Dumas, J.E. (1989). Attentional problems in dysfunctional mother-child interactions: an interbehavioral model. *Psychological Bulletin, 105*, 116-30.

214. Wells, K.C., Epstein, J.N., et al. (2000). Parenting and family stress treatment outcomes in attention deficit hyperactivity disorder (ADHD): an empirical analysis in the MTA study. [see comment] *Journal of Abnormal Child Psychology, 28(6)*, 543-53.

215. Pelham, W.E., Wheeler, T., et al. (1998). Empirically supported psychosocial treatments for attention deficit hyperactivity disorder. *Journal of Clinical Child Psychology, 27(2)*, 190-205.

216. Luria, A. (1961). *The role of speech and the regulation of normal and abnormal behaviors.* New York: Liveright.

217. Abikoff, H., Gittelman, R. (1985). Hyperactive children treated with stimulants: is cognitive training a useful adjunct? *Archives of General Psychiatry, 42(10)*, 953-961.

218. Pelham, W., Waschbusch, D. (1999). Behavioral intervention in ADHD. In H.C. Quay and A. Hogan, *Handbook of Disruptive Behavior Disorders.* (pp. 255-278). New York: Plenum Publishing Corp.

219. DuPaul, G.J. and Eckert, T.L. (1997). The effects of school-based interventions for ADHD: A meta-analysis. *School Psychology Review, 26*, 5-27.

220. Anastopoulos, A.D., DuPaul, G.J., and Barkley, R.A. (1991). Stimulant medication and parent training therapies for attention deficit-hyperactivity disorder. *Journal of Learning Disabilities, 24*, 210-218.

221. Anastopoulos, A.D., Shelton, T.L., DuPaul, G.J., & Guevremont, D.C. (1993). Parent-training for attention-deficit hyperactivity disorder: its impact on parent functioning. *Journal of Abnormal Child Psychology, 21*, 581-596.

222. Abramowitz, A.J. and O'Leary, S.G. (1991). Behavioral interventions for the classroom: Implications for students with ADHD. *School Psychology Review, 20*, 220-234.

223. DuPaul, G.J. (1991). Attention deficit-hyperactivity disorder: Classroom intervention strategies. *School Psychology International, 12*, 85-94.

224. Abikoff, H. and Gittelman, R. (1984). Does behavior therapy normalize the classroom behavior of hyperactive children? *Archives of General Psychiatry, 41*, 449-454.

225. Fiore, T., Becker, E., and Nero, R. (1993). Educational interventions for students with attention deficit disorder: Issues in the education of children with attentional deficit disorder [Special Issue]. *Exceptional Children, 60*, 163-173.

226. Sheridan, S.M., Dee, C.C., Morgan, J.C., McCormick, M.E., and Walker, D. (1996). A multimethod intervention for social skills deficits in children with ADHD and their parents. *School Psychology Review, 25*, 57-76.

227. Kolko, D.J., Loar, L.L., and Sturnick, D. (1990). Inpatient social-cognitive skills training groups with conduct disordered and attention deficit disordered children. *Journal of Child Psychology and Psychiatry and Allied Disciplines, 31*, 737-748.

228. Hinshaw, S.P., Buhrmester, D., and Heller, T. (1989). Anger control in response to verbal provocation: Effects of stimulant medication for boys with ADHD. *Journal of Abnormal Child Psychology, 17*, 393-407.

229. Cunningham, C. and Cunningham, L. (1995). Reducing playground aggression: student-mediated conflict resolution. *The ADHD Report, 3*, 9-11.

230. Hinsahw, S.P., Owens, E.B., et al. (2000). Family processes and treatment outcome in the MTA: Negative/ineffective parenting practices in relation to multimodal treatment. *Journal of Abnormal Child Psychology, 28(6)*, 555-68.

231. Epstein, J., Conners, C.K, Erhardt, D., Arnold, L.E., Hechtman, L., Hinshaw, S.P., Hoza, B., Newcorn, J.H., Swanson, J.M., Vitiello, B. (2000). Familial aggregation of ADHD characteristics. *Journal of Abnormal Child Psychology, 28(6)*, 595-9.

232. Fonagy, P., Target, M. (1994). The efficacy of psychoanalysis for children with disruptive disorders. *Journal of American Academy of Child and Adolescent Psychiatry. 33*, 1073-1086

233. Pelham, W.E., Carlson, C.L., Sams, S.E., Vallano, G., Dixon, M.J. & Hoza B. (1993). Separate and combined effects of methylphenidate and behavior modification on boys with attention deficit hyperactivity disorder in the classroom. *Journal of Consulting and Clinical Psychology, 61(3)*, 506-515.

234. MTA Cooperative Group. (1999). A 14-month randomized clinical trial of treatment strategies for attention deficit hyperactivity disorder. *Archives of General Psychiatry. 56*, 4555

235. Weiss, G., Hechtman, L. (1993). *Hyperactive children grown up: ADHD in children, adolescents, and adults.* New York: Guilford.

236. Hallowell, E. (1995) Psychotherapy of adult attention deficit disorder. In K. Nadeau, *A comprehensive guide to attention deficit disorder in adults.* (pp. 144-168). New York,: Brunner/Mazel

237. Hallowell, E., Ratey, J. (1994). *Driven to distraction.* New York: Pantheon.

238. Sussman, S., Ratey, N. (1995). *ADD coaching.* Lafayette Hill, PA: National Coaching Network.

239. Weiss, M., Hechtman, L., et al. (1999). *ADHD in adulthood: A guide to current theory, diagnosis, and treatment.* Baltimore, MD: The Johns Hopkins University Press.

240. Nadeau, K. (1994). *Survival Guide for College Students with ADD or LD.* New York: Magination Press.

241. Quinn, P. (1994). *ADD and the College Student.* New York: Magination Press.

242. Kratter, J. (1983). The use of medication in the treatment of attention deficit disorder with hyperactivity. *Dissertation Abstracts International, 44*, 1965.

243. Bemporad, J.R. (2001). Aspects of psychotherapy with adults with attention deficit disorder. *Annals of the New York Academy of Sciences, 931*, 302-9.

244. Parker, J.D.A., Sitarenios, G., and Conners, C.K. (1996). Abbreviated Conners' Rating Scales revisited: A confirmatory factor analytic study. *Journal of Attention Disorders, 1*, 55-62.

245. Conners C.K., Sitarenios G., Parker J.D., Epstein J.N. (1998a). The revised Conners' Parent Rating Scale (CPRS-R): factor structure, reliability and criterion validity . Journal of Abnormal Child Psychology, *26 (4)*, 257-268.

246. Achenbach, T.M. & Edelbrock, C. (1983). *Manual for the child behavior checklist and revised child behavior profile.* Burlington, VT: University of Vermont Department of Psychiatry.

247. DuPaul, G.J. (1991). Parent and teacher ratings of ADHD symptoms: Psychometric properties. *Clinical Child Psychology, 20*, 245-253.

248. DuPaul, G.J. & Barkley R.A. (1992). Situational variability of attention problems: Psychometric properties of the Revised Home and School Situations Questionnaires. *Journal of Clinical Child Psychology, 21(2)*, 178-188.

249. McBurnett, K., Swanson, J., Pfiffner, L., and Tamm, L. (1998). A measure of ADHD-related classroom impairment based on targets for behavioral intervention. *Journal of Attention Disorders, 2*, 69-76.

250. Achenbach, T. and Edelbrock, C. (1987). *Manual for the child behavior checklist — Youth self-report.* Burlington, VT: University of Vermont Department of Psychiatry.

251. Kovacs, M. (1993). *The Children's Depression Inventory (CDI),* Toronto: Multi-Health Systems, Inc

252. Reynolds, W.M. (1987). Reynolds adolescents depression scale in school age children. *ACTA Paedopsychiatry, 46*, 305-315.

253. Beck, A.R., Steer, R.A., Brown, G.K. (1996). *Beck Depression Inventory-II.* San Antonio: Psychological Corporation.

254. Corkum, P.V. and Siegel, L.S. (1993). Is the Continuous Performance Task a valuable research tool for use with children with attention-deficit-hyperactivity disorder? [see comments]. *Journal of Child Psychology & Psychiatry, 34*, 1217-39.

255. Epstein, J., Conners, C., Erhardt, D., March, J., and Swanson, J. (1997). Asymmetrical hemispheric control of visual-spatial attention in adults with attention deficit hyperactivity disorder. *Neuropsychology, 11*, 467-73.

256. Barkley, R.A., Grodzinsky, G., and DuPaul, G.J. (1992). Frontal lobe functions in attention deficit disorder with and without hyperactivity: A review and research report. *Journal of Abnormal Child Psychology, 20*, 163-188.

257. Shue, K.L. and Douglas, V.I. (1992). Attention deficit hyperactivity disorder and the frontal lobe syndrome. *Brain and Cognition, 20*, 104-124.

258. Ross, P.A., Poidevant, J.M., and Miner, C.U. (1995). Curriculum-based assessment of writing fluency in children with attention-deficit hyperactivity disorder and normal children. *Reading & Writing Quarterly: Overcoming Learning Difficulties, 11*, 201-208.

259. Teicher, M.H. (1995). Actigraphy and motion analysis: new tools for psychiatry. *Harvard Revue of Psychiatry, 3*, 18-35.

260. Biederman, J., Newcorn, J., and Sprich, S. (1991). Comorbidity of attention deficit hyperactivity disorder with conduct, depressive, anxiety, and other disorders [see comments]. *American Journal of Psychiatry, 148*, 564-77.

261. Spencer, T., Biederman, J., and Wilens, T. (1994). Tricyclic antidepressant treatment of children with ADHD and tic disorders. *Journal of the American Academy of Child & Adolescent Psychiatry, 33*, 1203-4.

262. Wozniak, J., Biederman, J., Kiely, K., Ablon, J.S., Faraone, S.V., Mundy, E., and Mennin, D. (1995). Mania-like symptoms suggestive of childhood-onset bipolar disorder in clinically referred children [see comments]. *Journal of the American Academy of Child & Adolescent Psychiatry, 34*, 867-76.

263. Andrulonis, P.A. (1991). Disruptive behavior disorders in boys and the borderline personality disorder in men. *Annals of Clinical Psychiatry, 3*, 23-26.

264. Elia, J., Stoff, D.M., and Coccaro, E.F. (1992). Biological correlates of impulsive disruptive behavior disorders: attention deficit hyperactivity disorder, conduct disorder, and borderline personality disorder. *New Directions For Mental Health Services. 54*, 51-7

265. Hinshaw, S.P. (1994). *Attention deficits and hyperactivity in children.* Thousand Oaks, CA: Sage.

266. Faraone, S.V. and Biederman, J. (1997). Do attention deficit hyperactivity disorder and major depression share familial risk factors? *Journal of Nervous and Mental Disorders, 185*, 533-41.

267. Alpert, J.E., Maddocks, A., Nierenberg, A.A., O'Sullivan, R., Pava, J.A., Worthington, J.J., 3rd, Biederman, J., Rosenbaum, J.F., and Fava, M. (1996). Attention deficit hyperactivity disorder in childhood among adults with major depression. *Psychiatry Research, 62*, 213-9.

268. Famularo, R., Fenton, T., Kinscherff, R., and Augustyn, M. (1996). Psychiatric comorbitity in childhood post traumatic stress disorder. *Child Abuse and Neglect, 20*, 953-961.

269. Arnold, L.E., Abikoff, H.B., Cantwell, D.P., Conners, C.K., Elliott, G., Greenhill, L.L., Hechtman, L., Hinshaw, S.P., Hoza, B., Jensen, P.S., et al. (1997). National Institute of Mental Health Collaborative Multimodal Treatment Study of Children with ADHD (the MTA): Design challenges and choices. *Archives of General Psychiatry, 54*, 865-70.

270. Pelham, W. and Gnagy, E. (1995). Summer treatment program for children with ADHD. *The ADHD Report, 3.*

271. National Institute of Health (1998). *NIH Consensus Statements: 110. Diagnosis and treatment of attention deficit hyperactivity disorder.* Bethesda, MD: National Institute of Health

272. Arnold, L.E., Abikoff, H.B., Cantwell, D.P., Conners, C.K., Elliott, G., Greenhill, L.L., Hechtman, L., Hinshaw, S.P., Hoza, B., Jensen, P.S., et al. (1998). *14-month randomized clinical trial of treatment strategies for attention deficit hyperactivity disorder.* Presentation at American Academy of Child and Adolescent Symposium. Oct, 1998. Anaheim, CA.

273. Pfiffner, L.J., Calzada, E., et al. (2000). Interventions to enhance social competence. *Child & Adolescent Psychiatric Clinics of North America, 9(3)*, 689-709.

274. Arnold, L.E., Chuang, S., et al. (2004). Nine months of multicomponent behavioral treatment for ADHD and effectiveness of MTA fading procedures. *Journal of Abnormal Child Psychology, 32(1)*, 39-51.

275. Conners, C.K., Epstein, J.N., et al. (2001). Multimodal treatment of ADHD in the MTA: An alternative outcome analysis. *Journal of the American Academy of Child & Adolescent Psychiatry, 40(2)*, 159-67.

276. Hinshaw, S.P., Owens, E.B., et al. (2000). Family processes and treatment outcome in the MTA: Negative/ineffective parenting practices in relation to multimodal treatment. *Journal of Abnormal Child Psychology, 28(6)*, 555-568.

277. Jensen, P.S., Hinshaw, S.P., et al. (2001). ADHD comorbidity findings from the MTA study: comparing comorbid subgroups. *Journal of the American Academy of Child & Adolescent Psychiatry, 40(2)*, 147-58.

278. March, J.S., Swanson, J.M., et al. (2000). Anxiety as a predictor and outcome variable in the multimodal treatment study of children with ADHD (MTA). *Journal of Abnormal Child Psychology, 28(6)*, 527-41.

279. Owens, E.B., Hinshaw, S.P., et al. (2003). Which treatment for whom for ADHD? Moderators of treatment response in the MTA. *Journal of Clinical Psychology, 71(3)*, 540-52.

Index

We Want Your Opinion!

Comments about **Attention Deficit Hyperactive Disorder**:

_____

_____

_____

_____

_____

Other titles you would like Compact Clinicals to offer:

_____

_____

_____

_____

To be placed on our mailing list, please provide the following:

Name: _____

Address: _____

_____

_____

E-mail: _____

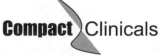

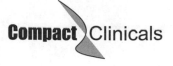

Order in 3 easy steps:

▶ 1   Provide complete billing and shipping information

Name _____   Company_____

Profession_____   Dept./Mail Stop_____

Street Address/P.O. Box_____

City/State/Zip_____

Telephone_____   ☐ Ship to Residence   ☐ Ship to Business

▶ 2   Choose Titles

For Clinicians:	Qty.	Unit Price	Total
Attention Deficit Hyperactivity Disorder *The latest assessment and treatment strategies*		$16.95	
Bipolar Disorder *The latest assessment and treatment strategies*		$16.95	
Borderline Personality Disorder *The latest assessment and treatment strategies*		$16.95	
Conduct Disorders *The latest assessment and treatment strategies*		$16.95	
Depression in Adults *The latest assessment and treatment strategies*		$16.95	
Obsessive Compulsive Disorder *The latest assessment and treatment strategies*		$16.95	
Post-Traumatic and Acute Stress Disorders *The latest assessment and treatment strategies*		$16.95	

For Physicians:

Bipolar Disorder: Treatment and Management		$18.95	

Continuing Education credits
available for mental health professionals.
Call 1-800-408-8830 for details.

Subtotal	
Tax (In MO ONLY, add 7.975%)	
Shipping ($3.75 first book/ $1.00 per additional book)	
TOTAL	

▶ 3   Choose Payment Method

Please charge my: ☐ Visa   ☐ MasterCard   ☐ Discover   ☐ American Express   ☐ Check Enclosed

Account # ___ ___ ___ ___ — ___ ___ ___ ___ — ___ ___ ___ ___ — ___ ___ ___ ___   Exp. Date ___ ___ / ___ ___

Name on Card _____   Cardholder Signature _____

Postal Orders: Compact Clinicals, 7205 NW Waukomis Dr., Suite A, Kansas City, MO 64151

Telephone Orders: Toll Free 1-800-408-8830   **Fax Orders:** 1(816)587-7198